Feminism and COVID-19

How Women Fare in the Face of a Global Crisis

edited by Julia Smith and Clare Wenham

The MIT Press
Cambridge, Massachusetts
London, England

The MIT Press
Massachusetts Institute of Technology
77 Massachusetts Avenue, Cambridge, MA 02139
mitpress.mit.edu

The MIT Press would like to thank the anonymous peer reviewers who provided comments on drafts of this book. The generous work of academic experts is essential for establishing the authority and quality of our publications. We acknowledge with gratitude the contributions of these otherwise uncredited readers.

This book was set in Stone Serif and Stone Sans by Westchester Publishing Services. Printed and bound in the United States of America.

Library of Congress Cataloging-in-Publication Data

Names: Smith, Julia, 1982– editor | Wenham, Clare editor
Title: Feminism and COVID-19 : how women fare in the face of a global crisis / edited by Julia Smith and Clare Wenham.
Description: Cambridge, Massachusetts : The MIT Press, [2026] | Includes bibliographical references and index.
Identifiers: LCCN 2025011050 (print) | LCCN 2025011051 (ebook) | ISBN 9780262554039 paperback | ISBN 9780262385695 pdf | ISBN 9780262385701 epub
Subjects: LCSH: COVID-19 Pandemic, 2020–2023—Social aspects | COVID-19 (Disease)—Social aspects | Women—Social conditions—21st century | Emergency management—Social aspects | Equality
Classification: LCC RA644.C67 G428 2026 (print) | LCC RA644.C67 (ebook)
LC record available at https://lccn.loc.gov/2025011050
LC ebook record available at https://lccn.loc.gov/2025011051

10 9 8 7 6 5 4 3 2 1

EU Authorised Representative: Easy Access System Europe, Mustamäe tee 50, 10621 Tallinn, Estonia | Email: gpsr.requests@easproject.com

Contents

1 Introduction

Julia Smith and Clare Wenham

Infectious disease outbreaks affect men, women, transgender, and nonbinary people in different ways.[1] This can range from sex-based differences in health outcomes, whereby physiological or hormonal characteristics may mean that infection with a pathogen leads to poorer outcomes in one sex than another, or these differences may be gendered. Gendered differences tend to appear as secondary effects of the policies introduced by governments to mitigate the spread of an infectious disease outbreak. These include, among other things, the impacts of changes to social interaction, paid and unpaid care work, and access to healthcare services.

As researchers who have previously researched the gendered effects of epidemics both individually and collectively, in January 2020, we anticipated a range of gendered effects related to COVID-19. We started to have conversations about the ways we thought people of different genders would be adversely and differentially affected by the emerging disease, initially considering those in China, where the pandemic began. Even back then, without the knowledge base we have since developed, we predicted that women would be most of the healthcare workers on the front lines of the response. We knew that the mass school closures in China and Hong Kong in January and February 2020 would have a knock-on effect on women, who suddenly had to provide round-the-clock childcare and home schooling to their children, either alongside their paid employment or sacrificing paid employment to do so.

Further cognizant of intersectional feminist thought, we knew not all women would be affected equally or in the same ways—race, class, geographies, socioeconomic status, and beyond, shaped further by neoliberal and colonial systems of oppression, would differentiate experiences. For example, we knew that the large foreign domestic worker labor force in Hong Kong almost exclusively comprises poor immigrant women of color working in often white, Western households, and they do so to send money back to their families in their home country. These women would face challenges if borders, which had suddenly closed as an emergency response measure for disease containment, remained restricted and they were not able to return to their families and/or to work. We also had major concerns about the physical security of women who were in lockdown in Wuhan and the likely impact this would have on violence against women (Wenham, Smith, and Morgan 2020). Drawing on the thinking of transnational feminist scholars (for example, Swarr and Nagar 2010; Fernandes 2013; Kaplan and Grewal 2002), we understood that the global pandemic response would be shaped by dominant approaches, primarily based on a Western neoliberal worldview, and that women's experiences of the pandemic would reflect not only these global inequities but their local realities. Similarly, resistance to the continued exploitation of women's labor and lack of concern for their security would both emerge from local efforts and foster global solidarities across geographies and cultures.

While we started to have these conversations among friends and colleagues, we also published a comment in *The Lancet*, and serendipitously, given the author limitations, we were required to dub ourselves the Gender and COVID-19 Working Group. Within a matter of days, we were being contacted by other researchers, policymakers, and activists from around the world (several of whom are now authors within this edited volume) wanting to join this group and work together to get much-needed recognition for the pandemic's emerging downstream effects on women and equity-deserving groups and to support policymakers by delivering the evidence they needed on these differential effects to be able to make decisions amid the crisis. This working group, chiming a cord with transnational feminism and activism, grew and grew over the course of the pandemic to over six hundred members, each sharing their research, their evidence needs, and their experiences as practitioners, creating a vibrant community of practice to respond to the gendered effects of COVID-19.

At the same time, we were fortunate enough to receive funding from the Canadian Institute of Health Research (CIHR) and from the Bill and Melinda Gates Foundation to continue to undertake research to document and analyze the gendered effects of COVID-19. Using a case study approach, this book provides a comprehensive summary of the work that this research team has produced over the course of the pandemic. Overall, the aim is to share how the pandemic and the response to it were lived by diverse women in multiple contexts, illuminating both unique experiences and shared solidarities across geographies and cultures.

The research team is multicentered, multidisciplinary, and transnational, covering case studies from Bangladesh, Brazil, Canada, China, the Democratic Republic of Congo, Hong Kong, Kenya, Nigeria, and the UK. The research team included members with backgrounds in international relations, anthropology, economics, agriculture, social policy, public policy, gender, and beyond. Zoom calls at all times of day and night fostered strong bonds of friendship, feminist allyship, and academic partnership. Despite disciplinary and methodological differences, we centered on wanting to provide evidence to improve the experience of a pandemic for women, whomever those women were and whatever hardships they were experiencing, and to do so as feminists, placing feminist principles at the core of our work together and our research outputs. We sought to contribute further to notions of transnational feminist activism through our interaction and desire to document and analyze the unequal impacts of the pandemic on those women made most vulnerable and shine a light on this for policymakers to understand the secondary effects of their decisions.

COVID-19

The COVID-19 pandemic is understood to have originated in Wuhan, China, in December 2019 and rapidly spread around the world. The World Health Organization (WHO) determined it a public health emergency of international concern (PHEIC) in January 2020. By March 2020, many countries had followed China's lead in implementing strict lockdowns, requiring populations to shelter at home, closing all but essential businesses and services, and restricting travel. As cases fell, by June 2020, most countries began to reopen their economies. Over the subsequent years, which saw varying waves of disease transmission around the world, countries responded through a variety of public health, socioeconomic, and travel measures. These ranged from zero-COVID approaches, embodied in strict lockdown and quarantine policies aimed at completely halting transmission at borders in contexts such as China and Hong Kong, to more balanced containment approaches weighing contagion alongside economic interests in contexts such as the UK and Canada. In most places, severe illness and death occurred among the elderly and those with underlying health conditions. However, these factors do not appear to determine who is susceptible to the long-term physical effects of COVID-19; an estimated 5 to 20 percent of those infected have longer-term health complications (known as "long COVID"). The introduction of mRNA vaccines by late 2020 and their subsequent mass rollout in high-income countries reduced the severity of illness in most cases. However, vaccine apartheid prevented most low-income countries from accessing vaccines as well as other technologies, in real time. At the time of this writing (May 2024), there have been approximately 775 million COVID-19 cases and over 7 million COVID-19-related deaths around the world (Our World Data in 2024).

Gender in Health Emergencies

Gender norms and experiences are determined by the society in which individuals interact. Gender is shaped by social, economic, and physical interactions in the health, justice, education, law, security, and industry sectors, which in turn influence how we understand social interactions and how individuals interact in societies. Intersectional feminist thinking emphasizes that gender is just one social location—reflective of systems of power and oppression—that shapes the inequities one does or does not experience and cannot be understood in isolation from other identities, such as those related to race and class (Bowleg 2021). Disaggregated data on sex, age, and disability will not on their own reveal the social norms and stereotypes that dictate how different populations respond to public health measures and lockdown orders. A health emergency places stress on preexisting inequalities and discrimination; it can initiate and compound multiple inequalities and discrimination, including those related to gender (Sharma et al. 2020). Rapid research into gender as well as ethnicity, disability, age, and economic experiences during health emergencies is vital to identifying the healthcare measures, social support, and protection needed to ensure public health compliance and equitable recovery, and yet it is often lacking.

While recognizing the need for intersectional approaches that consider gender in relation to other social positions, we ground this book—due to the focus on the experiences of women—within the growing literature on gender and health emergencies specifically. Emerging research has begun to demonstrate the downstream gendered effects of health emergencies prior to the COVID-19 pandemic. This includes the widespread analysis of the gendered effects of HIV/AIDS, which not only directly affected people of specific genders (men who have sex with men in many Northern contexts and women in sub-Saharan Africa) but also has had downstream effects on access to sexual and reproductive healthcare (Gruskin et al. 2017; Tariq and Kasadha 2022); on unpaid care burdens for women, particularly elderly women who take on the care of orphaned children (Ogden, Esim, and Grow 2006; Mannel et al. 2019); and on intimate partner violence (Dunkle and Decker 2013). Research on the HIV/AIDS response also illuminates women's central role as healthcare workers, community volunteers, and activists for rights-based responses (Cattaneo et al. 2019). Women living with HIV/AIDS, particularly in the Global South, have challenged global health organizations and funders to take gender seriously (Smith 2017).

Despite the recognition of the gendered effects of HIV/AIDS, this learning has not been transferred when it comes to other health crises. During the Ebola outbreak in West Africa (2014–2016), Harman (2016) noted the lack of gendered considerations in the response to the epidemic at all levels and highlighted the increasing presence of the "conspicuously invisible" woman within health-related decision-making. Women were involved in meetings, were put on task forces, and were encouraged to support the response to the epidemic, but within these fora, they lacked the power to implement decisions. Those decisions, in turn, lacked gender considerations. This situation reflected the longstanding critiques of representation politics from feminist research.

Zika, a mosquito-borne virus that emerged in Brazil in 2015 and manifested in children born with congenital Zika syndrome, demonstrated the tension between two aspects: women were instrumentalized on the front covers of newspapers to spur a securitization narrative demonstrating that women were at risk of infection, and in turn this would risk the health of their unborn children, while governments absolved themselves of responsibility to actually provide any needed support to the affected women. Women were told to clean their houses to prevent mosquito proliferation and to not get pregnant so as not to have a child born with Zika, but such messaging failed to consider the lived reality of those most at risk of infection. These were notably the poorest women in Brazilian society, shaped by the deep inequities created by rapid urbanization and capital flows, who were unable to afford air conditioning, those who work outside with greater exposure to mosquitos, and who were predominantly black or of mixed ethnic backgrounds (Wenham 2021).

In reviewing this past literature, we became acutely aware that where gender has been considered in health emergency response and literature, it has often been in simplistic ways, focused primarily on the experiences of women as a homogenous group, compared to men (usually also presented as a homogenous group) (Hankivsky and Kapilashrami, 2020). While data on sex and gender and COVID-19 are patchy around the world, data on race, (dis)ability, and socioeconomic status are simply nonexistent in most contexts, complicating intersectional analysis. Indeed, while writing this introduction, we were frequently dismayed by the lack of data on women of color, those living with disabilities, and variables of socioeconomic status. Similarly, prominent tools documenting the COVID response, such as United Nations (UN) Women and the United Nations Development Programme (UNDP)'s COVID-19 Global COVID-19 Response Tracker focused on policies seen to primarily effect women, including violence against women and women's participation in the workforce, with no similar tools considering how racial, socioeconomic, or other inequities were addressed in pandemic responses. These gaps in literature and data restrict the transformative potential of research on gender and public health emergencies, with this book aiming to contribute to filling this gap through a transnational focus that includes in-depth case studies based on diverse groups of women's lived experiences. Still, we note that much more needs to be done in terms of both intersectional data collection and outputs related to health emergencies.

Our Approach

Recognizing the limits of past research—including our own—on gender and health emergencies, we aim here to advance scholarship by building on the feminist political economy and global health security literature toward integrated transnational and intersectional feminist approaches.

Feminist political economy approaches illustrate that what and whom a society prioritizes during an emergency reveals the relationship in that society between ethics, politics, and power. Smith (2019) demonstrates that outbreaks follow a path dependency and that the tyranny of the urgent takes over the decision-making. According to Smith, the focus is centralized on epidemiology and public health decision-making, and the effects of the policies introduced from this public health perspective do not get considered amid the chaos of war on disease. A similar trend is identified by Davies and

Bennett (2016), who highlight that "structural issues are put aside in favor of addressing immediate biomedical needs." An emergent feminist global health security literature has sought to demonstrate that the state and the state-based structures of global health policy have made women's lives more insecure during pandemics (Wenham 2021). Moreover, having women on the ground who can deliver additional care, labor, and community support is of benefit to policymakers, who are often unable to fill this gap within state structures during a time of crisis. Thus, women become the solution to many policy challenges that emerge during a health emergency, while the threat of gender inequality remains ignored (Harman 2021).

While useful in understanding global processes, these approaches rarely recognize that these processes are not only gendered, but also racialized, class-based, and reflective of colonial traditions. Here, transnational feminism helps us understand the relationship between global structures and local lived realities, how patriarchal global health governance privileges some women over others, and the complexities of resistance. Transnational feminist thought has taken this analysis further to challenge Western models of white, classist understandings of feminism and integrates intersectional and postcolonial thought to demonstrate that colonial legacies and neoliberal economic and political systems, as well as other competing oppressions, shape the political and social order (Mohanty 2003).[2] Thus, it recognizes that women are not one category and that there is no one universal gendered experience, but that women's experience is further constrained by the state, race, class, sexuality, patriarchal and capitalist structures, and beyond, as well as understanding gender and agency in different ways (Enns, Comas-Diaz, and Bryant-Davies 2020). As this volume includes case studies from around the world, often focused on racialized and marginalized women, a transnational feminist approach enables a centering of these experiences, and it poses questions about relationships between these lived experiences with globalized systems of power.

Essential to these discussions is recognition that it is not possible to separate gender from other social locations or identities, as Western feminism has historically done. Intersectional feminism analysis, rooted in the praxis of African American feminism, challenges us to recognize intersecting systems of oppression and power and consider the complexities of how these relate to each other. Bowleg (2012) defines intersectionality as a theoretical framework "for understanding how multiple social identities such as race, gender, sexual orientation, SES, and disability intersect at the micro level of individual experience to reflect interlocking systems of privilege and oppression (i.e., racism, sexism, heterosexism, classism) at the macro social structural level" (p. 1267). The case studies in this book seek to illuminate how gender interacts with other social identities at the individual level to reflect the power relationships, inequities, and injustices in macrolevel pandemic responses. In this way we hope to contribute to advancing feminist global health scholarship.

We do so humbly, recognizing that as white, middle-class, educated editors in the Global North we are particularly cognizant of the meaningful differences between our experiences and those of our counterparts, both authors in this edited volume and, indeed, the women represented in this book. Thus, we have actively sought to engage with local feminist understandings and context in the individual chapters and have actively tried not to unify the themes and experiences of women worldwide but, rather, to construct each as "solidarities of difference" (Conway 2012). Following Mohanty (2003), we do not presume the existence of identical issue areas or priorities in considering the gendered impacts of COVID-19, as is evident through the variety of constituent groups and thematic considerations in this volume; however, we seek to identify interconnected themes that can support globalist activism and advocacy for policy change in the future.

Central Narrative

This book aims to contribute to the literature on the gendered implications of epidemics and pandemics through a case study approach that documents and analyzes the downstream gendered, and where possible intersectional, effects of the COVID-19 pandemic and of the national policies introduced in each case study country to mitigate COVID-19's spread. Despite the variety of cases and populations of women within them, we identify common themes, not necessarily of diverse women's experiences, but related to the globalized structures that shape them. We are cautious in expanding on these themes, recognizing the valid critiques of white Western feminism in seeking to generalize for women across the world who live in different contexts, with a range of intersectional considerations alongside that of gender. However, our case studies show that structural inequities pervading global systems and social structures, and those that limit women's public and private participation, create similar systems of power, oppression, and resistance, across our locations of study or "solidarities of difference" (Conway 2012).

Feminist scholarship from around the world has documented how, despite contextual differences, gender relations, meaning socially defined gender roles such as social reproduction, predispose women (and men) to perform certain roles within society. This is linked with social norms and gender stereotyping, which produce different understandings of what men and women should be doing within a community. Once these norms and their related predispositions become embedded within understandings of gender, women then perpetually perform social reproduction within the household, which means they have less time available for external opportunities and paid work. In turn, women become reliant on men's income, and the system perpetuates power and gender hierarchies. These gender hierarchies in turn create and promote institutions and structures that facilitate men's active participation in the public sphere and continue to maintain women in roles of unpaid care to facilitate men's capital production (Caprioli 2005). These roles generate women's economic dependency on men, reducing women's autonomy and creating opportunities for exploitation and violence.

As Galtung (1969) depicts, social, economic, political, legal, religious, and cultural structures and institutions at the global, state, and local level result in certain individuals and groups being unable to fulfil their basic needs or reach their full potential. Through these structures, power is exercised not only through coercive means but also through materials and ideas, with power relationships shaping the institutional and ideological formations where gender and intersectional identities and status are constructed. These inequities have direct impacts on individuals' livelihoods and wellbeing. Tickner (1992) writes of the "insecurity of individuals whose life expectancy was reduced, not by the direct violence of war, but by domestic and international structures of political and economic oppression." In this book, we are interested in how domestic and international responses to COVID-19 affected the insecurity many women live with due to structural oppression.

Building on such foundations, feminist approaches to global health security reorient health security away from protecting the state against external health threats to seeing the state (and related social and cultural structures) as a threat to or protector of the health of individuals (Davies and Harman 2020; Wenham 2021). These approaches further recognize that such structures have become globalized in tandem with the disproportionate power of corporate capital, which favors certain governance and cultural systems over others, as well as the increased pace and frequency at which people, information, and goods move around the world. Thus, we can ask, for example, not only how state health policy affects health outcomes, but how global capital flows perpetuate a global gender pay gap. While the answers will differ by contexts, and we note the variation of these, particularly considering intersectional and transnational differences among the women we study, we ask broad questions that apply across geographies and population groups. It is these common questions about how structural inequities shape women's experiences of the pandemic that tie these chapters together.

The chapters in this volume explore how dominant patriarchal structures were reflected in the response to the COVID-19 pandemic—and women's multiple and varied experiences of and resistance to these structures—across key themes. These themes were identified through an in iterative process of engaging with the broader literature on gender and health emergencies and the results from case study research. Some, such as unpaid care, cut across almost all chapters, while others are explored in depth within a specific chapter, such as chapter 10, on maternity and reproductive healthcare in the UK, and chapter 8, on community volunteer healthcare workers in Kenya. While the chapters that follow provide in-depth analyses of how these themes intersect with different contexts and interact with social positions beyond gender (such as race, ability, and economic position)—here, we sketch broad gender trends to situate the case studies within the global context.

Unpaid Care

Care is vital during a health emergency, and the ethics of care requires that we pay attention to the consequences of care arrangements—meaning the political ethics of giving and receiving care during a crisis. Feminist normative analysis is concerned with the arrangement of care structures, the distribution of labor, and the changing nature of care. Care represents a concrete activity but also a moral orientation. In an emergency there are those giving care, those instructing care, and those who are being cared for (Robinson 2016). Who is represented in each of these activities is a moral but also political decision that has implications for who has power over care.

Women with the least access to resources and who experience barriers to employment and services, such as those from ethnic minorities, are likely to bear the greatest unpaid care burdens. Race-based unpaid care gaps are apparent across the globe (i.e., the difference in the amount of time spent on unpaid care among different racial groups), often explained by the fact that racial and ethnic minorities are more likely to live in poverty, with less access to childcare or other support services (Women's Budget Group 2020). Women in the global south, those in rural regions, and those with lower education and low income also provide a disproportionate share of unpaid care (ILO 2018). In many contexts women of higher social economic standing outsource care work to other, less privileged, women, reinforcing inequities in access to employment and education.

Around the world, women do approximately three times more unpaid care work than men, performing 75 percent of such work globally (UN Women 2020). Women dedicate, on average, four hours and twenty-five minutes daily to care, while men's average is one hour and twenty-three minutes. Some 606 million women of working age perform unpaid care work on a full-time basis, compared with just 41 million men (UN Women 2020). This work includes childcare, care for elders and those who are ill or living with disabilities, cooking, and cleaning. Indeed, the amount of time women dedicate to unpaid care increases with the presence of children in the household (Dugarova 2020). Women are also usually responsible for the mental load of family and household management, such as scheduling activities and appointments. The economic contribution of unpaid care is roughly estimated at $10 trillion per year, around 13 percent of global GDP (ILO 2019). While the degree, type, and form of unpaid care varies greatly by context and social position—consider, for instance, the time difference between washing clothes with a washing machine and without one—what is consistent is that this work is usually done by women. This unequal distribution of unpaid care reflects the globalized norms and discriminatory social institutions that shape gender roles.

The COVID-19 response added to care burdens due to the closure of schools, childcare, and other services, as well as increased time spent on cleaning and household management. The average time spent on childcare around the world increased from twenty-six hours a week to thirty-one (UN Women 2020a). UN Women found that, in 2020, across thirty-eight countries, while both women and men experienced increased unpaid workloads, women did most of the care work. While men took on tasks such as shopping and helping with home schooling, women remained responsible for the cooking, cleaning, and overall childcare. Furthermore, parents report asking daughters for more help with care work than sons. COVID-19 also added to the intensity of unpaid care work, as new cleaning habits were developed to reduce risk and uncertainty related to the unfolding pandemic, and daily routines complicated family management. As health facilities restricted access or were avoided due to fear of infection, those in need returned home, where they were most likely to be cared for by women. In many countries, the majority of those who became seriously ill with COVID-19 were the elderly and were most likely cared for by women relatives and friends.

Increased unpaid care burdens come at a cost. The global trend of greater employment loss among women than men (discussed further below) has been linked to increased care responsibilities; with children home from school or facility-based care, women were unable to go to work. Increased unpaid care also generated increased anxiety as women tried to manage multiple and new tasks; in 2020, 70 percent of women participants in a Canadian survey reported increased anxiety and depression related to increased care work due to COVID-19 (Oxfam 2020). Chapter 10 in this volume, using quantitative data, points to a similar relationship between COVID-19-related care stressors and mental health. The qualitative chapters share the experiences of women saddled with increased unpaid care—including how these are shaped by structural inequities related to race, employment status, disability, and so on—and demonstrate both the effects on women's economic and personal security and their resilience and often unseen essential contribution to the COVID-19 response.

Paid Work

Around the world, women earn on average 16 percent less than men (UN Women 2020c). Black and Hispanic women earn on average the least, with white men earning the most (Kochhar 2023). The wage gap reflects a devaluing of the occupations most accessible to women due to gender and intersectionally biased norms, such as care professions and those that allow flexible hours to enable childcare. Most low-wage sectors, such as the service industry, are feminized in terms of both the workforce and the conditions of work. Feminized sectors see lower wages on average, often include greater precarity and less power over work conditions, and incur lower social status (Vosko, MacDonald, and Campbell 2009). Women of color or other ethnic minority groups disproportionately compose these lowest sectors of pay and highest sectors of precarity. Lower wages also reflect the motherhood penalty—the phenomenon wherein women who have children are less likely to earn the same as or more than men or women who do not (Benard and Correll 2010). Women, and particularly women of color, are also more likely to work in the informal sector, with 740 million working in the informal economy as market traders and domestic workers and in other occupations (Azcona et al. 2020). Informal work is often paid less and does not include the security or benefits associated with formal employment, making it particularly vulnerable during a crisis, such as the pandemic.

Feminized sectors in both the formal and informal economy—such as domestic work, the service industry, and tourism—were hardest hit by COVID-19-related closures and interruptions. Consequently, around the world, women lost the majority of jobs. An analysis of labor market data in 2020 by UN Women and the ILO found that, across fifty-five high- and middle-income countries, unemployment rates among women age twenty-five and up increased from 5.5 to 7.7 percent, compared to 4.7 to 7.1 percent among men during the first six months of the pandemic, and that more women (who are already less likely to be in the workforce) than men left the labor market altogether (twenty-eight million women age twenty-five and up, compared to 24.1 million men age twenty-five and up) (UN Women 2020b). Women in the informal sector were also affected, with incomes falling by 60 percent during the first month of the pandemic. Many of these losses were sustained, with women's employment recovery lagging behind men's almost everywhere in the world (Dhar and Mendina 2021). Such trends are partly attributed to continued impacts on feminized sectors, such as tourism, as well as ongoing unpaid care demands on women's time.

In this volume we provide nuanced, localized analysis of such global trends. Chapters 7, 8, and 4, on Kenya, Nigeria, and Canada, respectively, highlight how women's concentration in precarious employment resulted in heightened economic insecurity. Chapters 2 and 8, on Bangladesh and Nigeria, respectively, further emphasize how informal employment created barriers to accessing relief and supports. Chapter 10 presents quantitative data on employment and economic recovery across three case studies. While the degree of economic hardship varied greatly, each chapter charts a similar trend, and importantly, that trend is like the ones observed during previous health emergencies.

Violence against Women

Women bore the brunt of gender-based violence across geographies throughout the pandemic. As early as March 2020, advocates warned about the risks posed to women by globalized shelter-at-home orders, which required many women to isolate with their abusers without access to external support, as many service providers were forced to limit interactions or close to mitigate the spread of disease, as such public services were not considered to be essential (John et al. 2020). Data from the first months of the pandemic in Wuhan demonstrated a threefold increase in domestic violence during this time, and UK femicides related to domestic violence doubled in one month from March to April 2020 (Roesch et al. 2020).

Multiple researchers have tried to understand the extent to which violence against women has occurred and how this has changed during the pandemic compared to baseline. Data have included police data, calls to service providers, administrative data, and hospital data, each of which has its own limitations as to what it can or cannot say about the violence occurring. Calls to the police related to domestic violence rose in the UK and the US an estimated 6 percent during the first six weeks of the pandemic (Hsu and Henke 2020). However, it is likely that increases in domestic violence are considerably underreported, with people not wanting to seek external support both because of the risk of retaliatory violence and due to the pandemic. For example, when analyzing calls to domestic violence helplines, we see a much greater number of individual calls than that which is evident in police or other types of administrative data (Anderberg, Rainer, and Siuda 2022). Moreover, despite challenging data, rates of domestic violence are estimated to be 30 to 50 percent higher among Black, Hispanic, American Indian, and Alaskan native women in the US (CDC 2012). Data also show that sexual and gender minorities, women under the age of thirty, and women in rural locations are more likely to experience domestic violence than their counterparts (Kyriacou et al. 1999).

Additional variables have been evidenced to demonstrate who is most at risk of gender-based violence during the pandemic. Women who are in low-paid employment or who hold jobs in lower positions were at greater risk of violence (Colagrossi et al. 2022). Men were more likely to perpetuate violence if their economic position was affected by the social distancing measures brought in to prevent the spread of COVID-19 (Arenas-Arroyo,

Fernandez-Kranz, and Nollenberger 2021). Moreover, we can see changes in the way that women interacted with service providers: women were reporting to hospitals with much more serious conditions related to stages further along in the domestic violence abuse cycle than prior to the pandemic, presumably because they were following stay-at-home orders and did not want to interact with hospital facilities so as to avoid COVID-19 or not add to the burden of the healthcare system (Gosangi et al. 2021).

While working on this project, we made the conscious decision not to conduct research specifically on gender-based violence, recognizing that the complexity and ethical challenges of such work are outside the team's expertise. However, the topic frequently came up in interviews, with women wanting to share their experiences and perspectives, so these stories are included in some chapters (specifically, chapters 7 and 8 from Kenya and Nigeria, respectively). In addition, chapter 10 provides unique data on the incidence of conflict within households.

Health Care Workers

The operational response to the pandemic has been primarily carried out by women. Women are disproportionately employed in the healthcare sector. Some 70 percent of healthcare workers worldwide are women, along with up to 90 percent of social care workers globally, and women are particularly overrepresented in low-paid and underpaid healthcare jobs, such as nurses and social care workers. In many countries, women of color and Indigenous women are underrepresented in high pay/status positions in the health sector, such as physicians, but overrepresented in low pay/status positions such as care aids (Naqvi et al. 2022). The increasing reliance of high-income countries on healthcare workers from abroad (with little consideration of effects of this brain drain on low- and middle-income countries) has also increased the portion of migrant healthcare workers. However, while women have delivered on the care needs of large swathes of the population during COVID-19, they (particularly women of color and migrant women) have been underrepresented in decision-making positions during the pandemic.

This overrepresentation within the paid care economy has created important intersectional, gendered effects throughout the pandemic. COVID-19 infections among healthcare workers have disproportionately affected women, and racialized women more so than men (Miyamoto 2020).

Moreover, the lower-ranking and less-qualified and lowest-paid healthcare workers, the majority of whom are women, and often women of color, are more likely to have been redeployed into COVID-19-related care, meaning that their risk of infection is greater than those who are more highly skilled and paid (Chaudhry et al. 2020). Women healthcare workers in many contexts reported increases in violence, racism, discrimination and homophobia during the pandemic (Hennein et al. 2021; Smith et al. 2022; Lotta et al. 2021). At the same time, healthcare workers globally have criticized the ill-fitting nature of personal protective equipment (PPE) for women's body shapes, if women were able to access it in the first place.

The pandemic and its impact on the health system has had a knock-on effect on the workforce, with increased workloads across the sector, which has disproportionately affected women. This increased workload has had secondary effects on women's mental health and, indeed, their domestic care provision. For example, within the healthcare workforce, there have been higher rates of mental health concerns reported among women, particularly nurses, than men during the pandemic. This has manifested in depression, anxiety, insomnia, and distress (Lai et al. 2020). Being a woman, being a nurse, being infected with COVID-19, and having a child under ten years old have been shown to be key risk factors associated with increased mental health challenges (Mele et al. 2021). Gendered considerations have also become apparent in that health care workers have had to leave their children in childcare, while this provision was shut down for others, and in regard to the additional infection risks healthcare workers imposed on their households and dependents by working on the front line and then returning home or providing unpaid care to others. The mental health toll of this situation has been increasingly documented in qualitative research demonstrating the feelings of solitude, guilt, and added mental anguish experienced by healthcare workers who were already overburdened professionally (Smith et al. 2022). Chapters 5 and 7 in this volume provided further insight into the specific lived experiences of women healthcare workers in China and Kenya, a topic also touched on in chapter 6 on Hong Kong.

Mental Health

Even beyond the health workforce, women have been particularly impacted by mental health challenges during COVID-19, with higher reported levels of depression, anxiety, and other mental health problems. Prepandemic, women experienced depression and anxiety twice as often as men while experiencing more barriers to accessing care (Gadermann et al. 2021). Determinants of poor mental health among women include chronic environmental strain, pregnancy, and gender-based violence. For example, one in seven perinatal women experience increased anxiety, depression, and distress, with the risk being even higher among those experiencing a medically high-risk pregnancy (Fairbrother et al. 2017). The double burden carried by most women around the world—that of both unpaid care and paid employment—contributed to high levels of stress and feelings of failure. Those with poor mental health face employment barriers, may incur greater out-of-pocket health expenses, and face barriers to engaging in political and community processes. The disproportionate mental health burden women bear reinforces gender inequities and can be long-lasting.

The pandemic amplified the determinants of poor mental health among women, and it created new sources of anxiety related to potential exposure for healthcare workers. For example, a Canadian Mental Health Association survey found that the number of mothers reporting high levels of anxiety was twice that of other respondents (CMHA 2021). In the UK, women reporting underlying mental health issues increased from 11 percent to 27 percent during the first few months of the pandemic, with pregnant women particularly reporting increased anxiety (Petter 2020). In several of the chapters that follow, women describe declining mental health as a key effect of the pandemic on their well-being, identifying sources of stress and anxiety tied to increased unpaid care, financial insecurity, and frontline work. While this is by no means a mental health research project, we felt it was important to document the relationship between the social and economic effects of the pandemic on women and mental health. Chapters 2, 4, and 8 include such analyses.

Maternity Provision and Sexual Reproductive Health

COVID-19 also affected women's access to routine healthcare, and in particular, access to sexual and reproductive health services, including maternity care. We know that women's access to contraceptives is further determined by a range of intersectional factors relating to distance to provision, availability of disposable income, cultural context, and ability to negotiate sex. We presume, although there is not comprehensive data from 2020 onward, that each of these factors was intensified in many contexts. The range of social distancing measures, closures of nonessential public services, and widespread lockdowns had a knock-on effect on the production and distribution of contraceptives. This was further complicated by travel restrictions, meaning that routine global supply chains were disrupted, and consequently, many locations had to endure periods of time when they were unable to access contraceptives because of the pandemic (UNFPA 2020). Moreover, given the broader loss of income for many women across the world, those who routinely paid for contraception out of pocket also faced additional barriers in accessing it. The result of the combination of factors was an estimated 10 percent decline worldwide for short- and long-acting reversible contraceptive methods, with an estimated forty-nine million women with unmet needs for contraception and an estimated fifteen million unintended pregnancies (Riley et al. 2020).

Abortion access was also an issue of concern for women during COVID-19. For some women, access to abortion was cut off due to healthcare systems scaling back on all areas deemed nonessential, and the pandemic offered a window of opportunity for conservative administrations to further reduce women's access to termination. Other women had their access to abortion reduced because of travel restrictions, such as not being able to travel outside their neighborhoods, for example, or to travel internationally for those who live in restrictive settings. For others still, loss of employment and the financial challenges associated with the pandemic have prevented them from accessing abortion services. In contrast, some women experienced increased access to abortion provision as governments sought to liberalize such access, such as through permitting access to abortion at home and the increased use of tele-abortion (Moreau et al. 2021).

Maternity provision was also significantly affected by COVID-19 worldwide. As witnessed during the Ebola and Zika epidemics, the pandemic resulted in reduced utilization of ante- and postnatal care services. This was driven by both supply and demand—as with the provision of reproductive health services, ante- and postnatal care were seen as nonessential, and some healthcare providers resorted to being exclusively COVID-19 facilities. On the demand side, women avoided care due to fear of infection with COVID-19 in a healthcare setting or because they did not want to further burden health services in the midst of the pandemic. In some parts of the world, such services were replaced by video or phone calls with service providers, but in other parts of the world this just resulted in the suspension or reduction of services (Goyal et al. 2021). This reduction resulted in a reduced number of hospital and institutional births during the pandemic and fewer postbirth support services (such as lactation support). Given the data that demonstrate that Black and ethnic minority women disproportionately experience poorer outcomes utilizing maternity services (Dayo, Christy, and Habte 2023), we assume that such women will have been further put at risk during the pandemic.

This change to maternity provision has had a knock-on effect on women's experience of pregnancy, childbirth, and beyond, as well as outcomes. Women have reported feeling lonelier, being more afraid, and having limited information on how to care for themselves and their children, and they have suffered lower satisfaction with the experiences of pregnancy and of being a new parent compared to the prepandemic baseline. Modelers have sought to estimate the impact of this distortion on the healthcare system and have suggested that the changes to maternity care will result in an additional 1,157,000 infant deaths worldwide and an additional 56,700 maternal deaths (Roberton et al. 2020). While several case studies included pregnant women as research participants, the UK case study presented in chapter 9 specifically focuses on their experiences.

Approach and Methods

Early in the pandemic, the Gender and COVID-19 team developed the COVID-19 and gender matrix as a tool to assist us in conducting a systematic gender analysis (Morgan et al. 2021). A gender analysis matrix is a tool that seeks to systematically explore how gender-based power relations manifest to create inequities. In developing the gender and COVID-19 matrix, we started with recognized gender frameworks (see, for example, WHO 2011; JHPIEGO 2016) that identify how power relations manifest as inequities, including access to resources, roles and practices, norms and beliefs, decision-making and autonomy, and policies, institutions, and laws (Morgan et al. 2016). As these dynamics are multifaceted, gender domains allow for the identification of factors that could be used as proxies to better understand how gender-based power relations manifest. For topic-specific domains, we selected those known to be relevant for infectious disease transmission and control, including risk and vulnerability, illness and treatment, health systems and services, social and economic impacts, and security effects (WHO 2011). We then drafted questions for each cell, which were posed for further reflection and analysis related to the intersection of each topic-specific domain and gender analysis domain. For example, questions in the domain of risk and access to resources included "To what extent do men, women and gender minorities have access to knowledge about disease prevention?" and "To what extent do men, women and gender minorities have access to financial resources to purchase equipment and material needed to protect themselves from infection?" The focus was specifically on gender as a starting point, not end point, in the analysis.

During the initial stage of the project, each case study first aimed to explore such questions through literature and media scoping reviews, including search terms related to other intersectional inequities (race, income, and others) as appropriate for that context. We systematically searched national news, government and civil society sources, and academic literature to map which gendered effects were documented, and we analyzed these according to the domains of the matrix. The gender and COVID-19 matrix data are available online (www.genderandcovid-19.org), with findings from seven countries. The methodology underpinning the matrix approach has been documented in peer-reviewed papers (Smith et al. 2021; Morgan et al. 2021). While we utilized the same methodology across case study locations, the flexibility of the methodology aligned with transnational feminist approaches: from the initial country-level analyses using the matrix, we were then able to identify key contextual issue areas and the groups of women most affected in particular ways in each context, as well as gaps in the literature, which in turn directed our further research in diverse and differential ways. For example, the Canada matrix highlighted that immigrant women were particularly affected by structural inequities. In the UK, access to reproductive healthcare emerged as a key issue for women. Thus, the country-level matrices supported a tailored focus for each case study's research on contextually appropriate, specific topics and study populations.

In addition, the qualitative case studies, as well as the survey methods used in chapter 10, applied the matrix domains as a starting point, structuring questions around the topic themes and gender domains of the matrix. From this common starting point across the case studies, which was justified as a unified comparative research project, questions were then refined to be applicable to the local context and culture, recognizing that different social and political contexts and structures shape women's experience of crisis. Thus, we engaged with local feminist understandings and contexts to construct "solidarities of difference" across the chapters of the book, each of which has centered on a different population group, including our key thematic subjects as appropriate to that location and group of women. For example, many of the chapters focus on how gender roles structure women's responsibility to fill care deficits during crises and discuss how and why women experienced decreased personal security during COVID-19, recognizing that this was not just on account of gendered realities but that those most at risk were also those who inhabit multiple domains, including differing ethnic or racial groups, the lowest socioeconomic groups, or having disabilities, for example. Chapter 10, which engages survey results from three case studies, explores relationships between themes, such as the impact of increased care burdens on overall wellness. Other chapters focus on a specific theme: chapter 9, on the UK, specifically discusses access to maternal health services; chapter 5, on China, documents gender differences in the experiences of frontline workers. In this way, the gender and COVID-19 matrix provides the grounding framework for the transnational context and intersectional analysis that follows.

Qualitative Research Methodology

With the exception of chapter 10, which applies quantitative analysis to survey results across three countries, and chapter 11, which applies policy analysis to point the way to more gender-responsive pandemic planning, the chapters in this book draw on parallel qualitative research based on semistructured interviews. This approach is rooted in intersectional research approaches that, developing from Black feminism scholar activism in the US, aim to illuminate the lived experiences of marginalized groups (Cho et al. 2013). This includes a commitment to the creation of knowledge grounded in the experiences of people belonging to the groups most affected by the subject of the research, recognizing that knowledge is gained by acknowledging the specificity and uniqueness of lives rather than by simply adding or counting different groups of women (Yarrow and Pagan 2020). The chapters that follow focus on everyday life occurrences to capture both the ordinary and the extraordinary across a range of women who are in a shared situation—the COVID-19 pandemic—but are living it as subjective individuals in specific contexts (Sangster 1994). While recognizing that each case study and experience is unique, and indeed, while recognizing the intersecting determinants of women's lived experience during the pandemic, elements of commonality facilitate the analysis of clusters of shared experiences to illustrate recurring patterns and instances of struggle and empowerment (McIntosh and Wright 2019). The holders of these experiences, as those with intimate knowledge, are recognized as experts, particularly in terms of evaluating the effects of pandemic response on different groups of women. Such qualitative research adds meaningful inquiry based on the lived experiences of those most affected into health research and policy discussions (Sallee and Flood 2012).

Table 1.1 summarizes the semistructured interviews that were conducted within each case study. Our qualitative research approach did not entail collecting detailed demographic data, recognizing that such a process can be extractive and instead asking participants to share what information they were comfortable with and focusing on those intersecting identity factors that were most relevant to the context (McMillan et al. 2024). Furthermore, the case study approach employed in most chapters did not aim to provide population-representative samples but in-depth analysis of the lived experiences of particular groups of women, so table 1.1 reflects those groupings.

All data for both the qualitative and quantitative analyses were collected between March 2020 and March 2022. Each case study took its own approach to sampling and recruitment, as well as seeking ethics approval in their home country. Ethics approval for the overall project was provided by the Office of Research Ethics at Simon Fraser University in Canada. In most cases participants were recruited purposively through local networks and civil society groups, as well as advertisements, with some snowball sampling, as appropriate. Due to the physical distancing requirements of the pandemic, in some cases, interviews were held online or over the phone. In all cases, the authors of the chapters were directly engaged in data collection and analysis. Interviews were audio-recorded and then transcribed for analysis, using framework and thematic analysis approaches.

Scope and Limitations

This book is about women, which we define as anyone who identifies as such regardless of sex assigned at birth. We apply this broad definition recognizing that "women" is a socially constructed category defined by gender norms and roles that vary across contexts but that, within a globalized world, are shaped

Table 1.1
Qualitative research participants

Chapter and case study	Number of participants	Type of participants	Date of data collection
2—Bangladesh	40	28 women and 12 men living in urban slums	January to March 2021 and November 2021
3—Brazil	31	Women living in low- to middle-income urban outskirts	March to August 2021
4—Canada	26	20 racialized recent immigrant women and 6 representatives from civil society organizations	May to June 2020 and September to December 2021
5—China	11	8 women and 3 men first responders (healthcare workers, a scientist, and social workers)	December 2020 vto January 2021
6—Hong Kong	70	Women healthcare workers, low-income and precariously employed women, mothers, ethnic minority women	May to October 2020
7—Kenya	38	Women community health volunteers	April to June 2021
8—Nigeria	32	12 women living in urban slum communities, 8 informal women traders, 8 women living with disabilities	January to March 2021
9—UK	23	Pregnant women and new mothers	October to November 2020

by a dominant patriarchal narrative and a capitalist political economy. We recognize that the focus on women limits our analysis of structural inequities to their effects on this one gender. By no means do we mean to suggest that other genders have not also been affected by the COVID-19 pandemic in multiple ways, both similarly to and differently from what is presented here. We simply aim to focus our research questions on how one gender, across different contexts and social positions, has experienced the pandemic, providing one lens into how global structural inequities interact with health crises. We recognize that there is a need for research that documents the full range of gendered experiences of COVID-19, particularly those of people who identify outside the man-woman dichotomy, who are often rendered invisible. To this end, we recommend that readers also explore the work of Jarrett et al. (2020) and Restar et al. (2021) among others.

While we apply intersectional feminist approaches in recognizing that gender identity intersects with additional social positions related to race, sexuality, ethnicity, (dis)ability, and socioeconomic status and beyond, we did not collect full demographic data on participants, instead focusing on specific overlaps (such as adolescent girls or migrant women) that were relevant to each case study. Furthermore, while we explore how other social positions interact with gender to structure experiences, we also recognize that the primary focus on women's gendered experiences highlights specific experiences over others, which may overshadow other structural inequities and limits the analysis of these complexities (Mason 2019). Therefore, we encourage readers to seek out literature on race, (dis)ability, and other equity-based topics and COVID-19, as well as studies that apply intersectional approaches in detail, such as those by Laster, Pirtle, and Wright (2021) and Hankivsky and Kapilashrami (2020), among others.

As we do not understand gender to be a homogenous experience, the findings in this book do not seek to generalize about the constituent groups of women in each context. We recognize the limitations of a predominantly qualitative research project that focuses on subgroups of a population to illuminate the lived experience of these groups during the pandemic. However, we believe that our use of transnational feminist analysis and our observation of the gendered impacts of COVID-19 are illustrative and that this work evidences and provides deeper insight into the trends that have been experienced across temporalities and localities, demonstrating the broader phenomenon of the gendered effects of a pandemic globally.

Furthermore, as editors of this book, we recognized our positionality as white women based in high-income countries, working in privileged positions at well-resourced universities. We do not seek to universalize our own experience of gender and/or the COVID-19 pandemic. Thus, the country case study chapters in this book are all written by women living in and native to their respective contexts. The knowledge and expertise they bring to the chapters is notable. However, they also recognize that, as researchers based at universities or with civil society organizations, they too have a degree of privilege compared to the subjects of their research. This power imbalance structures research relationships. We have tried to recognize and mitigate this, as much as possible, by allowing women to share their experiences on their own terms (and in their own language) through a semistructured approach, compensating them for their time and ensuring free and easy access to researchers and results. We have left the quotes in this book verbatim, even when translated, to capture the voice of the women interviewed.

We also recognize that our relative power puts all of us at risk of the privilege hazard: "the phenomenon that makes those who occupy the most privileged positions among us—those with good educations, respected credentials, and professional accolades—so poorly equipped to recognize instances of oppression in the world" (D'Ignazio and Klein 2020). Our lived experience of privilege inhibits our ability to fully comprehend the experiences of others, particularly the harms they have experienced or might experience because of colonial, geographic, economic, and racial inequities, and to imagine possible solutions. We aim to mitigate this hazard, and to honor the experiences shared, by including participants' recommendations on how the challenges they experienced might be overcome in terms of both practical and immediate and longer-term systemic change. Chapter 11 specifically aims to provide guidance for a way forward toward improved gender-responsive pandemic preparedness, recognizing that with the privilege of compiling a book comes the responsibility to advocate for change. Through this book, we strive to amplify the voices of groups of women highly affected by the pandemic, by bringing their voices together and highlighting the strong areas of convergence, where possible, and divergence when important.

It is also important to note that we (editors and authors) are writing about an exceptional experience we also lived through as women. While our individual experiences are each unique and very different from those of the subjects included in the chapters, we also share a gendered experience of the pandemic structured by the same forces that imposed care work on women, restricted economic and physical autonomy, and distanced us from decision-making. Much of the research for this book was conducted while the authors simultaneously parented, due to childcare facility and school closures. Some of us had to navigate COVID-19 restrictions in healthcare systems while pregnant or ill. Others experienced COVID-19-related political unrest and insecurity. No doubt, these experiences shape the analyses that follow. We argue that these experiences, while important biases to acknowledge, are also a strength in that they enable a deeper understanding of the gendered nature of the pandemic.

Notes

1. We note that the research project from which this book was developed is focused on the gendered impacts on women exclusively. This is not to say that the gendered impacts on men, trans and nonbinary groups are not an important unit of analysis, but this is beyond the scope of our work.

2. Our project did not set out to undertake intersectional research, which we recognize was a design flaw of a project. However, the findings from our project were so overwhelmingly intersectional, we have demonstrated this across the case studies. However, because of the design and methods used, we do not think it is appropriate to designate this research as truly intersectional.

References

Anderberg, Dan, Helmut Rainer, and Fabian Siuda. 2022. "Quantifying Domestic Violence in Times of Crisis: An Internet Search Activity-Based Measure for the COVID-19 Pandemic." *Journal of the Royal Statistical Society, Series A (Statistics in Society)* 185 (2): 498–518. https://doi.org/10.1111/rssa.12780.

Arenas-Arroyo, Esther, Daniel Fernandez-Kranz, and Natalia Nollenberger. 2021. "Intimate Partner Violence under Forced Cohabitation and Economic Stress: Evidence from the COVID-19 Pandemic." *Journal of Public Economics* 194: 104350. https://doi.org/10.1016/j.jpubeco.2020.104350.

Azcona, Ginette, Bhatt Antra, Sara Davies, Sophie Harman, Julia Smith, and Clare Wenham. 2020. "Will the Pandemic Derail Hard-Won Progress on Gender Equality? Spotlight on Gender, Covid-19 and the SDGs." *UN Women*. https://eca.unwomen.org/sites/default/files/Headquarters/Attachments/Sections/Library/Publications/2020/Spotlight-on-gender-COVID-19-and-the-SDGs-en.pdf.

Benard, Stephen, and Shelley J. Correll. 2010. "Normative Discrimination and the Motherhood Penalty." *Gender & Society* 24 (5): 616–646. https://doi.org/10.1177/0891243210383142.

Bowleg, Lisa. 2012. "The Problem with the Phrase 'Women and Minorities': Intersectionality—An Important Theoretical Framework for Public Health." *American Journal of Public Health* 102 (7): 1267–1273.

Bowleg, Lisa. 2021. "Evolving Intersectionality within Public Health: From Analysis to Action." *American Journal of Public Health* 111 (1): 88–90. https://doi.org/10.2105/AJPH.2020.306031.

Caprioli, Mary. 2005. "Primed for Violence: The Role of Gender Inequality in Predicting Internal Conflict." *International Studies Quarterly* 49 (2): 161–178. https://doi.org/10.1111/j.0020-8833.2005.00340.x.

Cattaneo, Umberto, Margherita Licata, and Marcello Montefiori. 2019. *The Impact of HIV on Care Work and the Care Workforce*. Geneva: International Labour Organization.

CDC. 2012. *The National Intimate Partner and Sexual Violence Survey 2010–2012 Report*. Atlanta: Centers for Disease Control and prevention. https://www.cdc.gov/violenceprevention/pdf/NISVS-StateReportBook.pdf.

Chaudhry, Faisal B., Samavia Raza, Khurram Zeeshan Raja, and Usman Ahmad. 2020. "COVID 19 and BAME Health Care Staff: Wrong Place at the Wrong Time." *Journal of Global Health* 10 (2): 020358. https://doi.org/10.7189/jogh.10.020358.

Cho, Sumi, Kimberlé Williams Crenshaw, and Leslie McCall. 2013. "Toward a Field of Intersectionality Studies: Theory, Applications, and Praxis." *Signs: Journal of Women in Culture and Society* 38 (4): 785–810.

CMHA (Canadian Mental Health Association). 2021. "Summary of Findings Mental Health Impacts of COVID-19: Wave 2." CMHA. https://cmha.ca/wp-content/uploads/2020/12/CMHA-UBC-wave-2-Summary-of-Findings-FINAL-EN.pdf.

Colagrossi, Marco, Claudio Deiana, Andrea Geraci, and Ludovica Giua. 2022. "Hang Up on Stereotypes: Domestic Violence and an Anti-Abuse Helpline Campaign." *Contemporary Economic Policy* 40 (4): 585–611. https://doi.org/10.1111/coep.12571.

Conway, Janet. 2012. "Transnational Feminisms Building Anti-globalization Solidarities." *Globalizations* 9 (3): 379–393.

Davies, Sara E., and Belinda Bennett. 2016. "A Gendered Human Rights Analysis of Ebola and Zika: Locating Gender in Global Health Emergencies." *International Affairs* 92 (5): 1041–1060. https://doi.org/10.1111/1468-2346.12704.

Davies, Sara E., and Sophie Harman. 2020. "Securing Reproductive Health: A Matter of International Peace and Security." *International Studies Quarterly* 64 (2): 277–284.

Dayo, Elizabeth, Kayonne Christy, and Ruth Habte. 2023. "Health in Colour: Black Women, Racism, and Maternal Health." *Lancet Regional Health–Americas* 17: 100408. https://doi.org/10.1016/j.lana.2022.100408.

Dharr, Diva, and Rafael Diez de Medina. 2021. "Despite Recovery Efforts, Women's Unemployment Continues to Grow." Bill and Melinda Gates Foundation. https://www.gatesfoundation.org/ideas/articles/women-unemployment-covid19.

D'Ignazio, Catherine, and Lauren Klein. 2020. *Data Feminism*. Cambridge, MA: MIT Press.

Dugarova, Esuna. 2020. "Unpaid Care Work in Times of the COVID-19 Crisis: Gendered Impacts, Emerging Evidence and Promising Policy Responses." Paper presented at the UN Expert Group Meeting "Families in Development: Assessing Progress, Challenges and Emerging Issues. Focus on Modalities for IYF+30," New York, June 18, 2020.

Dunkle, Kristin L., and Michel R. Decker. 2013. "Gender-Based Violence and HIV: Reviewing the Evidence for Links and Causal Pathways in the General Population and High-Risk Groups." *American Journal of Reproductive Immunology* 69 (1): 20–26. https://doi.org/10.1111/aji.12039.

Enns, Carolyn Z., Lillian C. Díaz, and Thema Bryant-Davis. 2020. "Transnational Feminist Theory and Practice: An Introduction." *Women & Therapy* 44 (1–2): 11–26.

Fairbrother, Nichole, Allan H. Young, Areiyu Zhang, Patricia Janssen, and Martin M. Antony. 2017. "The Prevalence and Incidence of Perinatal Anxiety Disorders among Women Experiencing a Medically Complicated Pregnancy." *Archives of Women's Mental Health* 20: 311–319. https://doi.org/10.1007/s00737-016-0704-7.

Fernandes, Leela. 2013. *Transnational Feminism in the United States: Knowledge, Ethics, and Power.* New York: New York University Press.

Gadermann, Anne C., Kimberly C. Thomson, Chris G. Richardson, Monique Gagné, Corey Mcauliffe, Saima Hirani, and Emily Jenkins. 2021. "Examining the Impacts of the COVID-19 Pandemic on Family Mental Health in Canada: Findings from a National Cross-Sectional Study." *BMJ Open* 11 (1): e042871. https://doi.org/10.1136/BMJOPEN-2020-042871.

Galtung, Johan. 1969. "Violence, Peace, and Peace Research." *Journal of Peace Research* 6 (3): 167–191.

Gosangi, Babina, Hyesun Park, Richard Thomas, Rahul Gujrathi, Camden P. Bay, Ali S. Raja, Steven E. Seltzer, et al. 2021. "Exacerbation of Physical Intimate Partner Violence During COVID-19 Pandemic." *Radiology* 298 (1): E38–E45. https://doi.org/10.1148/radiol.2020202866.

Goyal, Manu, Pratibha Singh, Kuldeep Singh, Shashank Shekhar, Neha Agrawal, and Sanjeev Misra. 2021. "The Effect of the COVID-19 Pandemic on Maternal Health Due to Delay in Seeking Health Care: Experience from a Tertiary Center." *International Journal of Gynecology & Obstetrics* 152 (2): 231–235.

Hankivsky, Olena, and Anuj Kapilashrami. 2020. "Beyond Sex and Gender Analysis: An Intersectional View of the COVID-19 Pandemic Outbreak and Response. National Collaborating Centre for Determinants of Health." https://nccdh.ca/resources/entry/beyond-sex-and-gender-analysis-an-intersectional-view-of-the-covid-19-.

Harman, Sophie. 2016. "Ebola, Gender and Conspicuously Invisible Women in Global Health Governance." *Third World Quarterly* 37 (3): 524–541. https://doi.org/10.1080/01436597.2015.1108827.

Harman, Sophie. 2021. "Threat not Solution: Gender, Global Health Security and COVID-19." *International Affairs* 97 (3): 601–623. https://doi.org/10.1093/ia/iiab012.

Hennein, Rachel, Jessica Bonumwezi, Max Jordan Nguemeni Tiako, Petty Tineo, and Sarah R. Lowe. 2021. "Racial and Gender Discrimination Predict Mental Health Outcomes among Healthcare Workers beyond Pandemic-Related Stressors: Findings from a Cross-Sectional Survey." *International Journal of Environmental Research and Public Health* 18 (17): 9235. https://doi.org/10.3390/ijerph18179235.

Hsu, Linchi, and Alexander Henke. 2020. "The Effect of Social Distancing on Police Reports of Domestic Violence." *Feminist Economics* 27 (1–2): 362–379.

ILO (International Labour Organisation). 2018. *Care Work and Care Jobs for the Future of Decent Work*. Geneva: ILO.

Jarrett, Brooke A., Sarah M. Peitzmeier, Arjee Restar, Tyler Adamson, Sean Howell, Stefan Baral, and Sam W. Beckham. 2020. Gender-Affirming Care, Mental Health, and Economic Stability in the Time of COVID-19: A Global Cross-Sectional Study of Transgender and Non-Binary People. *medRxiv*. https://doi.org/10.1101/2020.11.02.20224709.

JHPIEGO (John Hopkins University Affiliate). 2016. "Gender Analysis Toolkit for Health Systems." JHPIEGO. https://gender.jhpiego.org/analysistoolkit/.

John, Neetu, Sara E. Casey, Giselle Carino, and Terry McGovern. 2020. "Lessons Never Learned: Crisis and Gender-Based Violence." *Developing World Bioethics* 20 (2): 65–68.

Kaplan, Caren, and Inderpal Grewal. 2002. "Transnational Practices and Interdisciplinary Feminist Scholarship: Refiguring Women and Gender Studies." In *Women's Studies on Its Own: A Next Wave Reader in Institutional Change*, edited by Robyn Wiegman, 66–81. New York: Duke University Press.

Kochhar, Rakesh. 2023. "The Enduring Grip of the Gender Pay Gap." Pew Research Center. https://www.pewresearch.org/social-trends/2023/03/01/the-enduring-grip-of-the-gender-pay-gap/.

Kyriacou, Demetrios, Deirdre Anglin, Ellen Taliaferro, Susan Stone, Toni Tubb, Judith A. Linden, Robert Muelleman, Erik Barton, and Jess F. Kraus. 1999. "Risk Factors for Injury to Women from Domestic Violence." *New England Journal of Medicine*. 342: 1892–1898. https://doi.org/10.1056/NEJM199912163412505.

Lai, Jianbo, Simeng Ma, Ying Wang, Zhongxiang Cai, Jianbo Hu, Ning Wei, Jiang Wu, et al. 2020. "Factors Associated with Mental Health Outcomes among Health Care Workers Exposed to Coronavirus Disease 2019." *JAMA Network Open* 3 (3): e203976. https://doi.org/10.1001/jamanetworkopen.2020.3976.

Laster Pirtle, Whitney N., and Tashelle Wright. 2021. "Structural Gendered Racism Revealed in Pandemic Times: Intersectional Approaches to Understanding Race and Gender Health Inequities in COVID-19." *Gender & Society* 35 (2): 168–179. https://doi.org/10.1177/08912432211001302.

Lotta, Gabriela., Michelle Fernandez, and Marcela Corrêa. 2021. "The Vulnerabilities of the Brazilian Health Workforce during Health Emergencies: Analysing Personal Feelings, Access to Resources and Work Dynamics during the COVID-19 Pandemic." *International Journal of Health Planning and Management* 36 (S1): 42–57. https://doi.org/10.1002/hpm.3117.

Mannell, Jenevieve, Samantha Willan, Maryam Shahmanesh, Janet Seeley, Lorraine Sherr, and Andrew Gibbs. 2019. "Why Interventions to Prevent Intimate Partner Violence and HIV Have Failed Young Women in Southern Africa." *Journal of the International AIDS Society* 22 (8): e25380. https://doi.org/10.1002/jia2.25380.

Mason, Corinne L. 2019. "Buzzwords and Fuzzwords: Flattening Intersectionality in Canadian Aid." *Canadian Foreign Policy Journal* 25 (2): 203–219. https://doi.org/10.1080/11926422.2019.1592002.

McIntosh, Ian, and Sharon Wright. 2019. "Exploring What the Notion of 'Lived Experience' Offers for Social Policy Analysis." *Journal of Social Policy* 48 (3): 449–467. https://doi.org/10.1017/S0047279418000570.

McMillan, John, Brian D. Earp, Wing May Kong, Mehrunisha Suleman, and Arianne Shahvisi. 2024 "The Wrong Word for the Job? The Ethics of Collecting Data on 'Race' in Academic Publishing." *Journal of Medical Ethics* 50 (3): 149–151.

Mele, Bria S., Jayna M. Holroyd-Leduc, Patricia Harasym, Sandra M. Dumanski, Kirsten Fiest, Ian D. Graham, Kara Nerenberg, et al. 2021. "Healthcare Workers' Perception of Gender and Work Roles during the COVID-19 Pandemic: A Mixed-Methods study." *BMJ Open* 11 (12): e056434.

Miyamoto, Inez. 2020. "COVID-19 Healthcare Workers: 70% Are Women." Daniel K. Inouye Asia-Pacific Center for Security Studies. https://dkiapcss.edu/nexus_articles/covid-19-healthcare-workers-70-are-women/.

Mohanty, C. (2003). *Feminism without Borders: Decolonising Theory, Practising Solidarity*. Durham, NC: Duke University Press.

Moreau, Caroline, Mridula Shankar, Anna Glasier, Sharon Cameron, and Kristina Gemzell-Danielsson. 2021. "Abortion Regulation in Europe in the Era of COVID-19: A Spectrum of Policy Responses." *BMJ Sexual & Reproductive Health* 47 (4): e14.

Morgan, Rosemary, Sara E. Davies, Huiyun Feng, Connie C. R. Gan, Karen A. Grépin, Sophie Harman, Asha Herten-Crabb, Julia Smith, and Clare Wenham. 2021. "Using Gender Analysis Matrixes to Integrate a Gender Lens into Infectious Diseases Outbreaks Research." *Health Policy and Planning* 37 (7): 935–941. https://doi.org/10.1093/HEAPOL/CZAB149.

Morgan, Rosemary, Asha George, Sarah Ssali, Kate Hawkins, Sassy Molyneux, and Sally Theobald. 2016. "How to Do (or Not to Do) . . . Gender Analysis in Health

Systems Research." *Health Policy and Planning* 31 (8): 1069–1078. https://doi.org/10.1093/heapol/czw037.

Naqvi, Habib, Reginald D. Williams, Owen Chinembiri, and Sam Rodger. 2022. "Workforce and Workplace Racism in Health Systems: Organisations Are Diverse but Not Inclusive." *Lancet* 400 (10368): 2023–2026. https://doi.org/10.1016/S0140-6736(22)02395-9.

Ogden, Jessica, Simel Esim, and Caren Grown. 2006. "Expanding the Care Continuum for HIV/AIDS: Bringing Carers into Focus." *Health Policy and Planning* 21 (5): 333–342. https://doi.org/10.1093/heapol/czl025.

Our World in Data. 2024. "17 Key Charts to Understand the COVID-19 Pandemic." https://ourworldindata.org/key-charts-understand-covid-pandemic.

Oxfam. 2020. "71 Per Cent of Canadian Women Feeling More Anxious, Depressed, Isolated, Overworked or Ill Because of Increased Unpaid Care Work Caused by COVID-19: Oxfam Survey." https://www.oxfam.ca/news/71-per-cent-of-canadian-women-feeling-more-anxious-depressed-isolated-overworked-or-ill-because-of-increased-unpaid-care-work-caused-by-covid-19-oxfam-survey/.

Petter, O. 2020. "One in Three Women Suffering from Loneliness in Lockdown." *Independent*, June 14, 2020. https://www.independent.co.uk/life-style/women/lockdown-loneliness-uk-gender-gap-women-a9565106.html.

Restar, Arjee J., Harry Jin, Brooke Jarrett, Tyler Adamson, Stefan David Baral, Sean Howell, and S. Wilson Beckham. 2021. "Characterising the impact of COVID-19 Environment on Mental Health, Gender Affirming Services and Socioeconomic Loss in a Global Sample of Transgender and Non-Binary People: A Structural Equation Modelling." *BMJ Global Health* 6 (3): e004424. https://doi.org/10.1136/bmjgh-2020-004424.

Riley, Taylor, Elizabeth Sully, Zara Ahmed, and Ann Biddlecom. 2020. "Estimates of the Potential Impact of the COVID-19 Pandemic on Sexual and Reproductive Health in Low-and Middle-Income Countries." *International Perspectives on Sexual and Reproductive Health* 46: 73–76.

Roberton, Timothy, Emily D. Carter, Victoria B. Chou, Angela R. Stegmuller, Bianca D. Jackson, Yvonne Tam, Talata Sawadogo-Lewis, and Neff Walker. 2020. "Early Estimates of the Indirect Effects of the COVID-19 Pandemic on Maternal and Child Mortality in Low-Income and Middle-Income Countries: A Modelling Study." *Lancet Global Health* 8 (7): e901–e908.

Robinson, Ruthie, and Cynthia Kellam Stinson. 2016. "Moral Distress: A Qualitative Study of Emergency Nurses." *Dimensions of Critical Care Nursing* 35 (4): 235–240.

Roesch, Elisabeth, Avni Amin, Jhumka Gupta, and Claudia García-Moreno. 2020. "Violence against Women during Covid-19 Pandemic Restrictions." *BMJ* 369: m1712. https://doi.org/10.1136/bmj.m1712.

Sallee, Margaret W., and Julee T. Flood. 2012. "Using Qualitative Research to Bridge Research, Policy, and Practice." *Theory into Practice* 51 (2): 137–144. https://doi.org/10.1080/00405841.2012.662873.

Sangster, Joan. 1994. "Women's History Review Telling Our Stories: Feminist Debates and the Use of Oral History." *Women's History Review*. 3 (1): 5–28. https://doi.org/10.1080/09612029400200046.

Sharma, Shreela V., Ru-Jye Chuang, Melinda Rushing, Brittni Naylor, Nalini Ranjit, Mike Pomeroy, and Christine Markham. 2020. "Social Determinants of Health-Related Needs during COVID-19 among Low-Income Households with Children." *Preventing Chronic Disease* 17: E119.

Smith, Julia. 2019. "Overcoming the 'Tyranny of the Urgent': Integrating Gender into Disease Outbreak Preparedness and Response." *Gender & Development* 27 (2): 355–369.

Smith, Julia, Lina Abouzaid, Joy Masuhara, Salima Noormohamed, Neli Remo, and Lynn Straatman. 2022. "'I May Be Essential but Someone Has to Look After My Kids': Women Physicians and COVID-19." *Canada Journal of Public Health* 113 (1): 107–116. https://doi.org/10.17269/s41997-021-00595-4.

Smith, Julia, Sara E. Davies, Huiyun Feng, Connie C. R. Gan, Karen A. Grépin, Sophie Harman, Asha Herten-Crabb, Rosemary Morgan, Nimisha Vandan, and Clare Wenham. 2021. "More than a Public Health Crisis: A Feminist Political Economic Analysis of COVID-19." *Global Public Health* 16 (8–9): 1364–1380. https://doi.org/10.1080/17441692.2021.1896765.

Swarr, Amanda. L., and Richard Nagar, eds. 2010. *Critical Transnational Feminist Praxis*. Albany, NY: State University of New York Press.

Tariq, Shema, Bakita Kasadha. 2022. "HIV and Women's Health: Where Are We Now?" *Women's Health* 18: 17455065221076341. https://doi.org/10.1177/17455065221076341.

Tickner, J. Ann. 1992. *Gender in International Relations: Feminist Perspectives on Achieving Global Security*. New York: Columbia University Press.

United Nations Population Fund (UNFPA). 2020. "UNFPA Supplies COVID-19 Update: 16 April 2020." https://www.unfpa.org/resources/unfpa-supplies-covid-19-update-16-april-2020.

UN Women. 2020a. "Whose Time to Care? Unpaid Care and Domestic Work During Covid-19." UN Women Data Hub. https://data.unwomen.org/sites/default/files/inline-files/Whose-time-to-care-brief_0.pdf.

UN Women. 2020b. "Explainer: Everything You Need to Know about Pushing for Equal Pay." UN Women, last modified February 22, 2024. https://www.unwomen.org/en/news/stories/2020/9/explainer-everything-you-need-to-know-about-equal-pay.

UN Women. 2020c. "Gender Equality: Women's Rights in Review 25 Years after Beijing." https://www.unwomen.org/en/digital-library/publications/2020/03/womens-rights-in-review.

Vosko, Leah, Martha MacDonald, and Iain Campbell. 2009. *Gender and the Contours of Precarious Employment.* Toronto: Routledge.

Wenham, Clare. 2021. *Feminist Global Health Security.* New York: Oxford University Press.

Wenham, Clare, João Nunes, Gustavo Correa Matta, Carolina de Oliveira Nogueira, Polyana Aparecida Valente, and Denise Nacif Pimenta. 2020. "Gender Mainstreaming as a Pathway for Sustainable Arbovirus Control in Latin America." *PLoS Neglected Tropical Diseases* 14 (2): e0007954. https://doi.org/10.1371/journal.pntd.0007954.

Wenham, Clare, Julia Smith, and Rosemary Morgan. 2020. "COVID-19: The Gendered Impacts of the Outbreak." *Lancet* 395 (10227): 846–848.

WHO. 2011. *Taking Sex and Gender into Account in Emerging Infectious Disease Programmes: An Analytical Framework.* Geneva: World Health Organization. https://iris.who.int/bitstream/handle/10665/207693/9789290615323_eng.pdf.

Women's Budget Group. 2020. "Crises Collide: Women and Covid-19. Examining Gender and Other Equality Issues During the Coronavirus Outbreak." Women's Budget Group. https://www.wbg.org.uk/wp-content/uploads/2020/04/Crises-Collide-Women-and-Covid-19.pdf.

Yarrow, Emily, and Victoria Pagan. 2020. "Reflections on Front-line Medical Work during COVID-19 and the Embodiment of Risk." *Gender, Work & Organization* 28 (S1): 89–100. https://doi.org/10.1111/gwao.12505.

2 Unbalanced Scales: Exploring the Impacts of the Unequal Burden of Responsibilities Borne by Women during the COVID-19 Pandemic in Dhaka, Bangladesh

Selima Sara Kabir, Moumita Islam, Amal Chowdhury, Nazia Mahmud, and Sabina Faiz Rashid

Introduction

The first COVID-19 case in Bangladesh was reported on March 8, 2020, and the first recorded death due to COVID-19 was on March 18, 2020. Up to August 2022, there were over 2 million confirmed cases of COVID-19 with 29,315 deaths in Bangladesh (World Health Organization 2022). The Ministry of Health and Family Welfare declared "general holidays" (effectively lockdowns) from March 24 to May 30, 2020, following the rising case numbers, in order to curb the spread (Mamun 2020). Following this, from 2020 to 2022, the government took a reactive approach to instituting lockdowns based on the number of cases and the global discourse around the different variants of COVID-19. Lockdowns led to public and private institutions (factories, shops, educational institutions, and so on) all being shut down and transportation restricted on the streets. While the first lockdowns in 2020 were strongly enforced, subsequent lockdowns were more relaxed and took a zonal approach, with high-infection areas facing stricter enforcement than others through 2021.

Bangladesh is the eighth most populous country in the world with 39.4 percent of the population living in Dhaka (UN 2022). Around 3.5 percent of the population migrate internally each year to cities, mostly due to climate change disasters or in search of employment (Parven et al. 2022). Although there are no exact estimates, the majority of informal-sector workers are domestic migrants living in urban slums (Mujeri 2020). According to the International Labor Organization (2013), around 87.5 percent of the labor force is employed in the informal sector. The formal labor force participation of women is 35 percent (World Bank 2022). Domestic work is one of the most common forms of informal work for women (Huq et al. 2021). Other common informal work includes street peddling and hawking, construction, and uncontracted work in factories. Moreover, women in Bangladesh are usually direct caregivers, looking after their husbands, children, and elders in the family (Chakraborty 2020). Women's roles in Bangladesh, particularly for poorer women with less agency, are limited to the private sphere. Even working women are expected to return home and then tend to the household (Chakraborty 2020).

As the capital city, and a site of rapid urbanization, Dhaka faces a massive influx of internal migrants from across the country. This results in growing income inequality evidenced by the stark differences in the living conditions of the upper and middle classes and the urban poor in Dhaka. Around seven million people of Dhaka's urban poor population reside in approximately 3,394 slums and are very crowded (Baser, Nahar, and Rahman 2021). According to a multiple indicator cluster survey in 2013, an average of 4.6 members (75 percent of slum households) live in one room (Bangladesh Bureau of Statistics 2015). Studies have found that a significant proportion of these households are female-headed; one study found that 53.5 percent of 387 households surveyed were female-headed. These women living in the slums often move to the city at great material cost to themselves and find themselves more vulnerable than their rural counterparts. This is due to the high cost of living, in addition to the poor living conditions in densely populated urban slums, where sanitation and drinking water facilities are shared between ten households (Rashid et al. 2020; Islam and Chowdhury 2022). Although piped water is available in certain slums, the supply is erratic and residents live in uncertainty about whether they will get water for drinking or washing. Maintaining isolation or distancing in the slum is not possible (Corburn et al. 2020; Hasan et al. 2021).

These difficult living conditions, combined with falling incomes, sudden wage losses brought about by the COVID-19 lockdown, and fears around the health risks of the virus impacted the mental and physical health of women living in slums (Rashid et al. 2020). Furthermore, life in the urban poor settlements of Dhaka only worsened following the lifting of the lockdown, and precariousness persisted well into 2021 and beyond. The incomes of urban slum dwellers were 42 percent lower than their incomes before the pandemic (BIGD n.d.). Informal-sector workers experienced a 49 percent drop in earnings along with continued food insecurity; 11 percent were not able to afford three meals a day (BIGD n.d.). In the case of urban poor women, 69 percent experienced a drop in income, and 47 percent of urban poor women took loans to cope; these figures come from a sample of 2,790 urban poor households in Dhaka slums (Rahman et al. 2020). These challenges compounded the existing global and local structural inequalities that had already placed women at a disadvantage (Madgavkar et al. 2020). Unsurprisingly, it was women—particularly the most marginalized groups of women, such as women heads of households—who were among the most affected by COVID-19 lockdowns (BIGD n.d.).

In this chapter, we aim to understand the unequal burden of invisible work shouldered by a subsection of women living in the urban slums of Bangladesh during the depths of the initial phases of the COVID-19 pandemic along with their subsequent interlinked challenges and the ways in which they navigated these responsibilities. In the following sections, we highlight these difficulties in detail through two major themes: financial and food insecurities and household burdens. Throughout this chapter, we explore the coping mechanisms employed by women to overcome the challenges they have faced.

Throughout, we consider how our diverse case stories highlight the heterogeneity of the lived experiences of urban poor women and how their experiences of the pandemic are shaped—as transnational feminist approaches emphasize—by not only physical location but also social locations such as economic class and marital status. This heterogeneity speaks to the need to avoid generalizations about such a large and growing population and to analyze these cases using an intersectional lens. This chapter affirms the critical importance of intersectional responses for future pandemics and other emergencies and that of catering to the worst-affected women among this already marginalized group. Stricken with poverty and family pressure, poor urban women had to shoulder the majority of their families' burdens—in terms of needs for food, financial obligations, chores, and more.

Methodology

For this study, we conducted one round of in-depth interviews over the phone (due to COVID-19 restrictions) from January 24 to March 10, 2021, with forty respondents (twenty-eight women and twelve men). These in-depth interviews focused on understanding the changes in household responsibilities for women, their coping mechanisms, and their financial and economic insecurities during the first phase of the lockdown from March to August 2020. These respondents were selected from the existing databases of slum respondents at BRAC University's James P. Grant School of Public Health, who had consented to their names and numbers being recorded, as well as from databases shared with us through our sister organization, BRAC, the world's largest NGO.

Following this, we purposively selected a cohort of fifteen respondents (twelve women and three men) from the original forty and conducted two further rounds of interviews in person (when conditions permitted) or over the phone from June to November 2021, depending on the COVID-19 situation.

This chapter draws on responses from respondents who lived in urban slums in Dhaka (Kallyanpur, Shyampur, Dholpur, and Agargaon) during the time of their first interview. The respondents varied in age from seventeen to fifty-five. Most of our respondents were married (nineteen), with nine widowed respondents, two unmarried respondents, and two divorcees. Among the participants, twenty-eight respondents had children and four did not. While nineteen respondents earned a monthly salaried wage (mostly domestic workers, some ready-made garment workers, drivers, and so on), four were daily wage earners, four owned their own business (three tea stalls and one computer repair shop), and the rest were not wage earners. In the rich tapestry of people living in Dhaka, these women would be on the fringes. They are disenfranchised and downtrodden in society and have to rely on each other within their own communities in order to survive.

Through this article, using a gender-centric critical medical anthropology framework, we look at how women were triply burdened. The framework utilizes an intersectional lens and tries to understand the cross-cutting factors of patriarchal and Bangladeshi cultural values against a backdrop of the social barriers linked to poverty and the structural violence of living in a slum.

Financial and Food Insecurities

The pandemic and resultant lockdown caused a huge upheaval in the lives of all our respondents as the economy came to a halt. During this time, the poor, already living precariously, became poorer, as they were unable to find alternative means of income. At this point, household members reported having to stretch out weekly rations for over a month.

> Yes it was very difficult. They gave 5 kg rice. How long would that last? They also gave oil, potatoes and lentils. Some gave all that, soap, mask and everything. This food did not last. We of course faced difficulty. We had to face a lot of difficulty, a lot of problems. There were times when we couldn't cook anything for five or six days. We didn't even have any work. Neither my husband nor me. (forty-six-year-old, public restroom cleaner, married, mother of two)

The government and certain nongovernmental organizations rolled out various stimulus and relief packages to support families impacted by job loss and reduced income during COVID-19. Many of these were targeted toward daily wage earners and those working in factories, which were shut during lockdown (UNICEF Bangladesh 2020). The government introduced twenty-five support measures (eighteen new interventions and seven expansions of existing programs) in 2020 and early 2021 to address the increasing precarity following lockdown (Bhattacharya and Hossain 2021). The total value of these programs has been estimated to be 1,250 billion taka; 60 percent of this valuation was reallocated from the fiscal year 2020, and the remaining 40 percent was earmarked for fiscal year 2021 (Bhattacharya and Hossain 2021).

However, according to respondents, the relief and stimulus check roll-out was inadequate and irregular. In certain cases, respondents referred to corruption and mismanagement of resource allocation, but in most cases, there just was not enough relief to go around. One public restroom cleaner mentioned that they had only enough from the relief materials to last their household of four for one week, and they had to sustain the amount with greatly reduced consumption to make it last for a month. Such experiences correspond with reports that due to weak governance, many households only received one installment of relief throughout the entire first rigid lockdown period of two months (Mujeri 2020).

While a few respondents were lucky and their landlords allowed them the flexibility to delay or even skip rent payments for a month, for most, their food expenses did not shrink with their income. Many respondents expressed fear of starvation as the lockdown was extended every few weeks and people were uncertain on how long it would continue. A thirty-year-old garment worker, who lost her husband to a work accident in 2014, had been working to raise her twelve-year-old son alone. She painfully recollected that no one in her family, either her own family or her in-laws, gave any form of financial, social, or mental support.

> When I could not eat, then I used to feel extremely sad. My son used to cry for food, used to tell me, "Mother I want to eat this or that," then I used to feel pain. I could not work, so I could not feed him or myself. (thirty-year-old garment worker, widow, mother of one)

A concern linked very closely to starvation was that all the women interviewed felt deeply responsible for their children's and family's well-being. Any discussion related to food and support was very closely linked to fear of and guilt about not being able to put food in front of their family. They worried not only about their children but also about their parents and extended family members. Speaking to these women, we found that they tend to prioritize others' needs, health, and well-being more than their own. Respondents spoke about losing weight and experiencing loss of energy and exhaustion from these worries as well.

> I have become thin due to overthinking about my parents, not so much for my children. How will they live or eat, what if they die. What happens to me. I still think about them. I am concerned about my father. He is bedridden. My mother can still walk. (thirty-five-year-old cleaner, widow, mother of one)

Women often skipped meals and prioritized their children.

> My son is small, so he needs a little because he eats little. Then sometimes we used to divide equally or give my husband more, and I ate less. (twenty-three-year-old Tea—stall manager, married, mother of two)

This respondent went on to explain that since her husband worked hard outside the home to earn money for the family, he needed more food than her: "I eat less because he is a young man; he stays outside more or eats more than me."

Another form of coping was food-sharing. A thirty-year-old respondent working as a domestic worker and raising two young children shared that her husband used to drive a bus for school but lost his job during the lockdown. She noted:

> Today I had nothing to cook so my *bhabi* (neighbor) has given me eggplant and pieces of Hilsha fish. And if she needs something or runs out of something she'll ask me the next time. (thirty-year-old domestic worker, married, mother of two)

Even though they were struggling with money, they were hopeful for better days to come.

Other respondents shared similar experiences. Women were very concerned about the practicalities represented by the loss of income due to the pandemic. They were concerned about food insecurity and took immediate, proactive measures to ensure that they were able to shop for food and feed their families.

Many respondents took out loans (formal and informal) to survive this difficult period. This added to the anxiety around having to pay back these loans on top of facing reduced income or no income at all. A housemaid shared that in the slums, money lenders and others who were willing to loan cash often trusted women more than men. This, too, was rooted in the realities of women being less mobile and, as it was commonly acknowledged, less likely to abscond with the money, disappear, or waste the money, while men had a reputation for spending borrowed money to buy cigarettes and drugs.

> Here in the slums, it is easier for the females to get the loans. And the males who are gamblers or drug addicts can get money if they pawn or sell something. (private car driver in his mid-to-late fifties [exact age unknown], married, father of three)

Aside from food insecurity, financial insecurity caused high levels of stress as well. After taking those loans, women often struggled with paying them back, which heightened their stress. During our second follow-up sessions around June 2021, more than half of our respondents shared that their financial worries had not lessened with the lifting of the lockdown and the declining numbers of COVID cases. They shared that even though they started working again, their income was lower than before the pandemic. This was around the time when they stopped receiving financial support from NGOs, other private organizations, and the government but still had to pay off debts.

Increased economic insecurity, lack of food, and unpaid debts often led to arguments and fights in the household. Three of our respondents shared that their husbands had physically beaten them. One domestic cleaner started crying while sharing that her husband had beaten her multiple times for cash that she did not have. She also stated that even though she faced domestic violence frequently, she could not even consider leaving him because of societal stigma and shame and, more importantly, because of their daughter.

> I think the males should take more responsibility. A female comes to her husband's home to have a well-off life, right? I have only been beaten at my husband's. I was better when I did not have my daughter . . . I have to worry about my daughter's future. Have to get her married. (domestic worker in her late thirties [exact age unknown], married, mother of two)

Domestic violence is one of the many sad realities of these urban poor women who continue to shoulder the maximum burden and often invisible trauma that comes with poverty in a city. This is corroborated by similar studies conducted by BRAC based on reports from their community-based women's groups (Polli Shomaj), which noted a 24 percent rise in reported incidents of gender-based violence in 2020 compared to 2019 (BRAC 2020). Unfortunately, women living in slums have been facing abuse since long before the COVID-19 pandemic, and it only became more pronounced during the pandemic.

Household Responsibilities: Increased Burden on Women

Out of our twenty-five women respondents, twenty-one women stated that the pandemic and the initial lockdown led to a multitude of challenges for them, including increased household work. However, in contrast, our seven men respondents typically cited their job loss as their main concern during lockdown and did not mention household chores. One of the specific questions we asked the men was regarding their contribution to the household during that time, and we similarly asked women if they received support from their husbands and sons. Based on the respondents' answers, it was rare for men to help around the house.

To understand the changes in the household responsibilities for women, we began by asking them about their daily routines prior to the pandemic. Responses illustrate that the conditions faced by women were not new, as they were already in charge of the cooking, cleaning, and child-rearing activities. In fact, in many cases, working women would return from work early to ensure that there was food on the table. However, findings show that the pandemic compounded an already uneven division of labor, as family members were at home due to school closures and restrictions on movement within the settlements. In slums, with family members confined to a room or home in poor households, which usually had a bed and little space for much else, this only added to the stress for women.

Households were expected to take extra precautions to keep COVID-19 infections at bay. Women had to collect water from the nearby taps more regularly, as well as wash clothes and clean the house more frequently and more intensively than before. This was more difficult in urban slums, where the water supply was erratic and only worked at certain hours, and all sanitation services—latrines and bathing and washing areas—were shared among numerous households. This required finding time to get chores done, as well as coordinating community schedules, which was stressful for women.

> During the lockdown, the work pressure increased. I had to boil water several times a day. I had to keep things clean a lot with soap and water and made sure everyone washed their hands. (forty-one-year-old domestic worker, married, mother of three)

Women's responsibilities were not limited to personal hygiene; they also had to ensure that their family members were taking necessary sanitary precautions. One of the men respondents mentioned that they would now wash the few clothes they owned daily, whether the clothes were dirty or not, as a COVID precaution. In this case, he was able to identify this, as he was the one doing the washing since his mother was sick and his wife was pregnant. Typically, these responsibilities were taken up by women so quietly that most of the men were not even aware of the increased burden in the household and saw it as part of women's responsibilities.

One housewife respondent noted the increased workload despite being the one managing the household work all by herself even before the COVID lockdown. Her husband was a rickshaw puller, and during the lockdown, he could not work anymore. She has two school-going children who were both at home. According to her, there was an increase in the amount of cooking food, washing clothes, and bringing water compared to the prepandemic situation. Even though the workload increased and her husband was home during the lockdown, she never asked for her husband's help, nor did he assist her. She said, laughing,

> Have you ever seen men working in the kitchen? Never! Even though now I have more pressure due to the lockdown, these jobs [cooking, washing, cleaning, and taking care of the house] are my responsibilities. I cannot ask my husband to do this. My mother, my mother-in-law never did this, how can I? (twenty-eight-year-old housewife, mother of two)

A common perception among men was that women's household work was far less difficult and not as important as the work they, themselves, did outside the home, which earns an income. A thirty-two-year-old tea stall owner, who lived with his wife and two-year-old son, described how household chores required less energy than having to earn an income. He also stated that household chores are a natural part of women's lives and this cannot be shared—a view in keeping with the gendered roles and expectations that are widely prevalent. Women have also internalized these gendered roles to the extent that they are not accustomed to seeing men helping out women in the kitchen or in general with typical daily household chores.

Men who did try to assist, particularly in the kitchen with cooking, felt very awkward. Closed kitchens shared by households were usually dominated by women who cooked and cleaned and caught up on their daily lives. It was embarrassing for men to be seen in the kitchen, and some of them said that men would be taunted by others if they cooked. One respondent, who does receive support from her husband, shared that she would try to dissuade him from entering the kitchen so others would not think poorly of her.

> I have told him that the other people might think that I force you to work and think bad of me. He'll say that whatever he does for me, he does it voluntarily. People will not know. (nineteen-year-old domestic worker, married, mother of one)

Even though the workload had increased substantially, most women never asked for help from their spouses or sons:

> Well, my daughter helped me out with tasks. Largely, I was the one who had to do everything. You know men, men cannot do household chores. They don't understand it. Cooking is a woman's job. (forty-one-year-old domestic worker, married, mother of three)

Only four out of twenty-five women gave a different type of response and shared that their husbands were very supportive and assisted with the increased household workload during the lockdown. For example, one twenty-three-year-old domestic worker said she felt less exhaustion and stress compared to other respondents because of her husband's assistance, such as heating food while she breastfed their young baby.

> Not everyone is the same. Many men think that females should cook. They think that we should cook them the food as they earn the money. But my husband loves me like that. (twenty-three-year-old domestic worker, married, mother of two)

However, when probed about the ways in which he assisted her, it did not seem to be very significant. She still woke up at 6 A.M. to ensure that she was able to finish the cooking, cleaning, and other household responsibilities on time. Even among the rare instances in which men provided support to their partners, we can see that these forms of support were often small and inconsistent and did not significantly reduce the burdens faced by the women. With many of our women respondents, household help from their husbands was typically limited to occasionally taking an active role in parenting. Many respondents (both men and women) noted that the one privilege of lockdown was being able to spend more time with their children.

Overall, the majority of respondents (twenty-nine out of forty) acknowledged that the overall household work pressure increased during the lockdown, which they found at times overwhelming and stressful. In the Bangladeshi cultural and social context, gendered roles and responsibilities persist and women are most likely to take on the responsibilities of household chores (Islam and Sharma 2021). Their constant labor in the house came with a significant impact on their health and well-being. Many respondents went through extreme mental distress due to the above-mentioned issues. Out of our respondents, twenty-nine (twenty-five women and four men) stated that their anxiety and distress had increased compared to their life before the pandemic. Most of our respondents shared that they regularly experienced stress and tension and that they remain often in an anxious state and feel sad, in addition to having trouble sleeping and experiencing a loss of appetite.

Women often came together to draw on mutual support as a coping strategy. One adolescent girl noted that she overcame feelings of vulnerability by chatting with her friends when she felt despair:

> Normally I do not talk much, but I often chat with my friends. . . . I can talk to aunty freely about anything. She's a really fun person. She can make me laugh a lot. She likes to *onek dustami kore* (fool around) sometimes she forgets she has to cook food while she's talking to me. She always gives me great advice when I am sad. (seventeen-year-old adolescent girl, lives with her grandmother)

Such quotes demonstrate that in addition to managing the practical challenges of feeding and caring for their families during the pandemic, women also provided each other with emotional support.

Discussion

Gender inequalities exist in urban poor settlements, as Bangladesh's culture upholds patriarchal values and beliefs that privilege and empower men. Even though it seems easy to paint these inequalities as black and white, the power dynamics that shape relationships between men and women are nuanced. Since numerous variables contribute to gender inequality, particularly in urban areas (such as cultural practices, conventional gender roles, social identities, poverty, systemic power inequalities, and discrimination in access to loans), it is important for us to consider a range of nuanced perspectives.

Indeed, we do not assume that all women interviewed had the same experience, and thus we have described a range of issues that were raised to us. Using the critical medical anthropology framework, we can explore how the added precarity of COVID-19 not only can be seen to exacerbate existing systemic challenges but made them more apparent.

Our findings demonstrate how women are expected to undertake family and household responsibilities. Being the primary caregivers, women faced increased household pressures during the first two years of the COVID-19 pandemic. During the lockdown, women's already invisible and unpaid household work increased, and it was especially pronounced in the urban slums of Dhaka (Islam and Chowdhury 2022). Typically, women's household responsibilities are thought to be balanced by men taking on the economic burdens as the "rice-winner" of the family. However, particularly during crisis, women often need to negotiate through the spaces thought to be reserved for men to ensure that the family is cared for. It was interesting to note that this division of labor among men and women in terms of the public (going out to earn) and the private (looking after the household) resulted in women having to undertake the burden of financial decision-making as well, given that food security was directly linked to financial security. This is a result of the inherited practice of urban informal settlement that prioritizes and appreciates men's and boys' contributions to public life and the workforce over women's contributions to unpaid domestic work, caregiving, and community service. This in turn means that even when women are contributing to earning wages and running the family, they are hardly given any recognition for this contribution.

The decisions that these women are forced to make—such as who should eat and who should survive on less food—speak more of the structural inequality that they live under rather than empowerment (Kabeer 1999). They themselves feel stuck making these decisions without any help from their partner or the state (Bhopal 1997). Women respondents expressed a strong sense of duty toward ensuring that their family is taken care of before considering themselves, as is common in South Asian cultures (Das and Kemp 1997). To them, this is very natural and nonnegotiable, so they worry about their parents, in-laws, siblings, and other family members (Morley and Crossouard 2016). Thus, even seemingly empowered steps toward financial decision-making, such as accessing credit, are steeped in internalized patriarchal notions of women's duty.

Such experiences illustrate that agency and empowerment are neither binary nor uniform; women do not either have or lack agency (Giddens 1987). Rather, even some of the most vulnerable and marginalized poor women enact agency by working within the systems that exist to ensure their own, and their families', welfare. The coping mechanisms adopted by respondents helped them to survive and push through immediate conditions. While these were not permanent solutions, they speak to the ways in which women negotiate within the patriarchal constraints put upon them. These women found ways to gather and help each other (by creating safe spaces to share emotions, food, and even money as necessary) at a time when everyone was feeling isolated and unsupported. These experiences echo Kandiyoti's (1988) work on bargaining with the patriarchy to find ways to survive and live despite the structural barriers of poverty.

Moreover, within the heteronormative framework, there is an increased likelihood that women are not given space to voice their anxiety (Gill and Orgad 2022). For example, while not all of our women respondents expressed that household chores were a burden, this does not mean they did not feel the increased stress of additional chores under lockdown; it is probable that they did not voice this distress because, within our patriarchal society, women are not given the space to do so, or they felt oppressed by other issues more strongly (Morley and Crossouard 2016). Oftentimes, because of their internalized patriarchal norms, urban poor women may not realize that their stress is a result of these chores or even consider that they are experiencing stress.

Conclusion

The women respondents included in this study demonstrated resilience in terms of pushing through the COVID-19 pandemic and taking care of themselves and their families despite the unfairness of the systemic challenges they face. It is important to reflect on their experiences and for the government and policymakers to address the underlying causes of gender inequalities.

The women we interviewed are consistently denied equal access to social and economic opportunities and services due to structural inequalities. These constantly practiced inequalities between men and women initially seem to have both immediate and longer-term impacts on women, which place them in vulnerable situations when crises, such as the COVID-19 pandemic, unfold. This vulnerability ultimately negatively affects the whole of society as well as the pandemic response itself. Reducing gender disparities will create societies that are more resilient in the face of crisis.

References

Bangladesh Bureau of Statistics. 2015. *Multiple Indicator Cluster Survey 2012–2013*. Bangladesh: UNICEF. https://www.unicef.org/bangladesh/en/reports/multiple-indicator-cluster-survey-2012-2013.

Baser, Shahadat, Shamsun Nahar, and M. Maksudur Rahman. 2021. "Inequality in Household Resources and Amenities in Dhaka City: The Case of Dhanmondi, Pallabi, and Kallayanpur." *Dhaka University Journal of Earth and Environmental Sciences* 9 (1): 49–62. https://doi.org/10.3329/dujees.v9i1.54861.

Bhattacharya, Debapriya, and Mursalin Hossain. 2021. "Unpacking the COVID-19 Stimulus Packages: The Devil Is in the Details." Centre for Policy Dialogue, May 28. https://cpd.org.bd/unpacking-the-covid-19-stimulus-packages-the-devil-is-in-the-details-debapriya-bhattacharya-and-mursalin-hossain/.

Bhopal, Kalwant. 1997. *Gender, "Race" and Patriarchy: A Study of South Asian Women.* London: Routledge.

BIGD (BRAC Institute of Governance and Development). n.d. "PPRC-BIGD COVID-19 Livelihoods & Recovery Panel Survey." BRAC Institute of Governance and Development. https://bigd.bracu.ac.bd/study/rapid-survey-on-immediate-economic-vulnerabilities-created-by-covid-19-and-the-coping-mechanisms-of-poor-and-marginal-people/.

BRAC. 2020. "Data Underscores that Gender-Based Violence Is Rising with COVID-19." BRAC, December 22. http://www.brac.net/latest-news/item/1298-.

Chakraborty, Shiney. 2020. "COVID-19 and Women Informal Sector Workers in India." *Economic and Political Weekly* (35): 17–21.

Corburn, Jason, David Vlahov, Blessing Mberu, Lee Riley, Waleska Teixeira Caiaffa, Sabina Faiz Rashid, Albert Ko, et al. 2020. "Slum Health: Arresting COVID-19 and Improving Well-Being in Urban Informal Settlements." *Journal of Urban Health: Bulletin of the New York Academy of Medicine* 97 (3): 348–357. https://doi.org/10.1007/s11524-020-00438-6.

Das, Ajit K., and Sharon F. Kemp. 1997. "Between Two Worlds: Counseling South Asian Americans." *Journal of Multicultural Counseling and Development* 25 (1): 23–33.

Giddens, Anthony. 1987. *Social Theory and Modern Sociology*. Cambridge, UK: Polity Press.

Gill, Rosalind, and Shani Orgad. 2022. "Get Unstuck!: Pandemic Positivity Imperatives and Self-Care for Women." *Cultural Politics* 18 (1): 44–63. https://doi.org/10.1215/17432197-9516926.

Hasan, Shaikh Mehdi, Susmita Das, Syed Manzoor Ahmed Hanifi, Sohana Shafique, Sabrina Rasheed, and Daniel D. Reidpath. 2021. "A Place-Based Analysis of COVID-19 Risk Factors in Bangladesh Urban Slums: A Secondary Analysis of World Bank Microdata." *BMC Public Health* 21 (1): 502. https://doi.org/10.1186/s12889-021-10230-z.

Huq, Lopita, Razia Sultana, Firoza Ashravee, and Nusrat Jahan. 2021. "Livelihood Transitions of Women Workers During COVID-19: The Case of Domestic Workers in Dhaka." BRAC Institute of Governance and Development (BIGD) Research Brief 9. https://opendocs.ids.ac.uk/opendocs/handle/20.500.12413/17284.

International Labor Organization. 2013. "Decent Work Country Profile." https://www.ilo.org/sites/default/files/wcmsp5/groups/public/@dgreports/@integration/documents/publication/wcms_216901.pdf.

Islam, Faisal Bin, and Madhuri Sharma. 2021. "Gendered Dimensions of Unpaid Activities: An Empirical Insight into Rural Bangladesh Households." *Sustainability* 13 (12): 6670. https://doi.org/10.3390/su13126670.

Islam, Moumita, and Amal Chowdhury. 2022. "Increased Burdens on Women in Bangladesh during the COVID-19 Pandemic." Gender and COVID-19 Project. https://www.genderandcovid-19.org/wp-content/uploads/2022/06/PAC00521_Gender-Covid-19-Evidence-Download-Bangladesh-002.pdf.

Kabeer, Naila. 1999. "Resources, Agency, Achievements: Reflections on the Measurement of Women's Empowerment." *Development and Change* 30 (3): 435–464. https://doi.org/10.1111/1467-7660.00125.

Kandiyoti, Deniz. 1988. "Bargaining with Patriarchy." *Gender and Society* 2 (3): 274–290. https://www.jstor.org/stable/190357.

Madgavkar, Anu, Olivia White, Mekala Krishnan, Deepa Mahajan, and Xavier Azcue. 2020. "COVID-19 and Gender Equality: Countering the Regressive Effects." McKinsey Global Institute. https://www.mckinsey.com/featured-insights/future-of-work/covid-19-and-gender-equality-countering-the-regressive-effects.

Mamun, Shohel. 2020. "Coronavirus: Bangladesh Declares Public Holiday from March 26 to April 4." *Dhaka Tribune*, March 23, 2020. https://www.dhakatribune.com/bangladesh/204680/coronavirus-bangladesh-declares-public-holiday.

Morley, Louise, and Barbara Crossouard. 2016. "Gender in the Neoliberalised Global Academy: The Affective Economy of Women and Leadership in South Asia." *British Journal of Sociology of Education* 37 (1): 149–168. https://doi.org/10.1080/01425692.2015.1100529.

Mujeri, Mustafa K. 2020. "Saving Informal Sector Workers from Pandemic Shock." *Financial Express*, August 20. https://thefinancialexpress.com.bd/views/views/saving-informal-sector-workers-from-pandemic-shock-1597944664.

Parven, Afshana, Indrajit Pal, Apichon Witayangkurn, Malay Pramanik, Masahiko Nagai, Hiroyuki Miyazaki, and Chanakan Wuthisakkaroon. 2022. "Impacts of Disaster and Land-Use Change on Food Security and Adaptation: Evidence from the Delta Community in Bangladesh." *International Journal of Disaster Risk Reduction* 78: 103119. https://doi.org/10.1016/j.ijdrr.2022.103119.

Rahman, Hossain Zillur, Narayan Das, Imran Matin, Mohammad Abdul Wazed, Shakil Ahmed, Nusrat Jahan, and Umama Zillur. 2020. "Livelihoods, Coping and Support During COVID-19 Crisis (Phase I)." BRAC Institute of Governance and Development. https://bigd.bracu.ac.bd/wp-content/uploads/2020/06/PPRC-BIGD-Final-April-Survey-Report.pdf.

Rashid, Sabina F., Bachera Aktar, Nadia Farnaz, Wafa Alam, Samiha Ali, Farzana Mansoor, Imran Hossain Mithu, Ateeb Ahmed, and Abdul Awal. 2020. "Impact of COVID-19 Lived Experiences of the Urban Poor in Slums during the Shutdown." BRAC James P. Grant School of Public Health (BRAC JPGSH). https://www.ariseconsortium.org/learn-more-archive/impact-of-covid-19-urban-poor-in-slums-shutdown-in-bangladesh/.

UNICEF Bangladesh. 2020. "Tackling the COVID-19 Social and Economic Crisis in Bangladesh: Providing Universal, Lifecycle Social Security Transfers to Protect Lives and Bolster Economic Recovery." UNICEF Bangladesh https://www.unicef.org/bangladesh/media/5256/file/%20Tackling%20the%20COVID-19%20economic%20crisis%20in%20Bangladesh.pdf%20.pdf.

UN (United Nations) Department of Economic and Social Affairs, Population Division. 2022. "World Population Prospects 2022." https://population.un.org/wpp/.

World Bank. 2022. "Labor Force Participation Rate, Female (% of Female Population Ages 15+)." https://data.worldbank.org/indicator/SL.TLF.CACT.FE.ZS?locations=BD.

3 "It Is the Woman Who Has to Do Everything, Paid or Unpaid": Work, Gender, and COVID-19 in Brazil

Mariela Rocha, Aponira Maria de Farias, Brunah Schall, Eduardo Ryo Tamaki, Paloma Porto, Paulo Silva Júnior, Flora Gonçalves, and Denise Nacif Pimenta

Introduction

Brazil experienced some of the highest numbers of COVID-19 cases and deaths per capita in the world. As of June 2022, official statistics had recorded 669,010 deaths, with 31,693,502 infected (Brazil Ministry of Health 2022). Deaths were particularly high among Black people, regardless of their age, their education level, or the socioeconomic level of the municipality where they lived (Batista et al. 2020), with deaths among Black women in the lowest-paid employment categories being the highest within this group (Prates et al. 2021).

In addition to the high number of deaths and infections, Brazil faced governance challenges between the federal, state, and municipal levels, often due to political-ideological differences. The federal government, led by President Jair Bolsonaro during the first two years of the pandemic, fostered an institutional "herd-immunity" strategy. The government disregarded infection prevention strategies, letting the disease spread rapidly through the population. It used slogans such as "It is not up to the State to take care of everyone," and "The suspension of economic activities kills more than the virus," as well as reinforcing the idea of "herd immunity by contagion" as a strategy to discredit social isolation measures and vaccination policies. This was a stark contrast to many governors, mayors, scientists, and health professionals committed to following WHO guidelines in fighting the disease. While the federal government advocated an approach that let the virus spread, the planning and execution of public policies to mitigate disease were left to local mayors and governors. This led to conflict between the federal and local governments, partially solved by the Supreme Court's decision to safeguard and ensure several protocols for the prevention and containment of infection (Ramos, Ramos, and Costa 2020). Ultimately, the federal executive was left with administrative decisions, while mayors and governors had the authority to manage the pandemic as they saw fit.

Federal government resistance to implementing emergency aid combined with the increases in the prices of fuel, cooking gas, and primary food items contributed to inflation. Concurrently, the federal government's employment-generating policies were ineffective. The Emergency Program for the Maintenance of Employment and Income (BEm) was established in April 2020 through law 14.020/2020:

> The objective of the program [BEm] is that the worker and the employer can make individual or collective agreements to reduce the working day, with a proportional reduction in the salary, or temporarily suspend the employment contract. During the period of the agreement, which cannot exceed 120 days, the Federal Government assumes part of the costs resulting from the suspension or reduction of the journey. (Instituto Brasileiro de Desenvolvimento, Jutiça e equidade [BRIDJE Institute] 2021)

This program proved insufficient to meet the needs of those most affected by the pandemic. For example, it did not include informal workers or self-employed professionals, which in the first quarter of 2022 corresponded to roughly 50.4 percent of the total number of people in the workforce (Fundo Brasil, 2022). Among these, 48.8 percent were women, and of those, 52.5 percent were Black women (Fundo Brasil 2022). In a previous assessment by Gênero e Número (2020a), more than four million women in Brazil were informal domestic workers who earned less than a minimum wage. This number corresponded to over 70 percent of the total number of women in the workforce (Gênero e Número 2020a). Furthermore, among Black women, 47.8 percent were informally employed (Gênero e Número 2020b).

Ultimately, the pandemic ravaged Brazil's economy, highlighting structural inequalities that had long been part of the country's history. In the last quarter of 2021, 35 percent of Brazilians were unemployed or underemployed (DIEESE 2022). In addition, the average income fell by 8 percent (DIEESE 2022), while inflation rose by 15.2 percent in just two years (between February 2020 and February 2022), leaving 33 million Brazilians hungry and 125 million facing food insecurity (PENSSAN Network 2022).

This chapter focuses specifically on the impact of COVID-19 on women dwelling in urban communities in Brazil, particularly asking how the pandemic affected their work and well-being. We take a broad view of work, including household and care labor, remote work, informal work, and precarious work. We consider the secondary effects of changes to work on women's well-being, and we assess government policies related to work through an intersectional gender lens. Our findings demonstrate that structural inequalities within Brazil made women's work, particularly that of racialized and low-income women from urban slum communities, vulnerable to the secondary effects of the pandemic. This in turn contributes to broader transnational feminist discussions, including those embedded in this volume, around how global capitalist structures and framings have influenced the gendered impacts of pandemic policy.

Women and Inequality in Brazil

Inequality is not new to Brazil, and neither is it unidimensional. According to the World Inequality Report, "In Brazil, the bottom 50% earn 29 times less than the top 10%" (Chancel et al. 2022, 14). This inequality has differing effects across society, including across genders. In Latin America, women who are married or in common-law marriages do nearly twice as much domestic work as their single counterparts (Nieto 2014). Women in Brazil dedicate up to twenty-one hours a week to household work, whereas men spend about eleven hours a week on the same tasks (Ribas 2021). This work remains largely invisible, due to the undervaluing of all tasks associated with care and maintenance in everyday life (Blanc, Laugier, and Molinier 2020). In the fields of both social reproduction and wage employment, women appear as the central protagonists in carrying out domestic care work—essential activities for society, whether in terms of reproduction or the well-being of its members (Guimarães and Hirata 2020). As primary caregivers, women are more exposed to illness in the professional and domestic spheres.

As we analyze the impact of COVID-19 on women, it is also necessary to look beyond gender, taking into consideration and articulating the multiple vulnerabilities to which women are exposed. Across gender lines, type of employment and income can either mitigate or amplify vulnerabilities, particularly those related to housing and food security, both challenges for the 16 percent of the population living in urban slums (World Bank 2018). Black women are overrepresented among those living in slums, as well as among those working in precarious employment. Akotirene (2020, 22) writes that in Brazil, "racism structured by modern colonialism insists on giving heavy burdens to black women." In Brazil, women (mainly Black women) make up 70 percent of the frontline healthcare workers that were combatting the pandemic (Wenham et al. 2022). Black women also experience poorer health outcomes and lower life expectancy than white women (Hogan et al. 2018). Nuanced analysis of women's experiences must take into consideration these additional equity dynamics.

Methods

Thirty-one in-depth interviews were carried out based on a semistructured script with women from low- to middle-income urban outskirts, sixteen in Cabana do Pai Tomás (Belo Horizonte, Minas Gerais) and fifteen in Sapopemba (São Paulo, São Paulo). The interviewees were women between twenty-three and sixty-four years old; 70.96 percent were Black, 45.16 percent were married or in common-law marriages, and 64.70 percent had children. Most interviewees reported low family income; 54.83 percent received up to two times the minimum wage a month, totaling 2,424 Brazilian reais, or 448.10 US dollars, a month. Interviews were conducted via phone from March to August 2021. Women were invited to participate in the research through previous contacts of the researchers with people from each location and then snowball sampling. Interviews were recorded, transcribed, and analyzed by thematic category, incorporating intersectionality in order to analyze not only the general experiences of women respondents, but how these were shaped by structural inequities related to gender, class, and race.

Results

Household and Care Labor

When asked about the impact of the pandemic on their load of unpaid household and care labor, most of the interviewees said there was a significant increase in work, mainly due to the sanitary measures brought in to reduce the spread of COVID-19, with more time spent at home preparing meals, helping children with schoolwork, and caring for elderly or sick family members. Most women reported that the responsibility for housework and care fell mainly on them:

I did the work, you know, there was no division. . . . It is the woman who is doing it, who is there . . . who has to do everything, paid or unpaid. (Brown woman,[1] thirty-two years old, Cabana do Pai Tomás, Belo Horizonte, Minas Gerais [MG])

The interviews reveal the burden of women's work during the pandemic, providing broader evidence of a care crisis in the country. In several interviews, women related this issue to the traditional gender roles they observe inside their families:

Some men don't care about it. They go to the bar, right? Go to the street. And the woman, they already have that thing about housework. (Brown woman, fifty years old, Cabana do Pai Tomás, Belo Horizonte, MG)

My brother doesn't do it (housework) because . . . I say it's a little bit of how we were raised, right? Because it used to be like this, for example: "It's the girl who has to do things, the boy doesn't do it." So this system was created. (Black woman, forty-two years old, Sapopemba, São Paulo, São Paulo [SP)

My mother and I are the women of the house, so we make the food, we clean the kitchen. Men at home don't have this perception, right? I don't know if they don't have it, but they have the perception that there will be someone to do it. So, consequently, whether we like it or not, we go on automatic, right? (Black woman, twenty-one years old, Sapopemba, São Paulo, SP)

We, who are women, are more concerned with the house, with children, with everything. Man, in my point of view, the vision of man I think is just working, putting food inside the house. (Brown woman, thirty-three years old, Sapopemba, São Paulo, SP)

In contrast to these reports made by Brown and Black women, all of whom defined themselves as unemployed or working in informal jobs, two white women with stable jobs and higher incomes said that household and care labor was equally distributed between them and other family members. One of them, who also has a higher educational level, emphasized that household tasks are a form of labor and therefore should be paid if not shared equally: "I usually tell my children, I'm not a maid, if they wanted me as a maid, they would have to pay me a salary" (white woman, thirty-nine years old, Sapopemba, São Paulo, SP),

The other associated the unconventional gender roles she was exposed to as a child with her building of an egalitarian division of labor in her family:

I come from a family where the father stayed at home with the daughters and took care of the house, and my mother worked. So here at home it's like this, everyone has to play a part for everyone to be okay. (white woman, thirty-eight years old, Sapopemba, São Paulo, SP)

Notably, these reports demonstrate the need to go beyond the gender variable when understanding COVID-19 experiences, as women even in the same territory had very different experiences depending on race, class, and educational level.

Beyond household labor, COVID-19 produced additional responsibilities for administering families' well-being (Teixeira 2020). With such a burden of activities and responsibilities domestically, many women were forced to leave their jobs—formal or informal—to dedicate themselves to family care:

> After my mother came out of intubation, she became dependent [on care], so I came to take care of her. So, I had to quit my job to come [home] to stay, and help take care of her. I don't even consider that what I'm doing is bad, because I should take care of my mother; it's more than my obligation. (Black woman, twenty-six years old, Cabana do Pai Tomás, Belo Horizonte, MG)

Here, the interviewee perceives care as something beyond her "own obligation," in the sense that it is her innate responsibility: to take care of her mother. This situation offers a real-world example of the broader phenomenon of domestic production and care responsibilities limiting women's participation in paid work, which in turn leads to a vicious circle of poverty (Abramo and Valenzuela 2016).

Remote Work

Women said that working from home completely changed their routines, as they faced the challenge of having overlapping tasks of paid and unpaid labor:

> We came to work remotely and remote work is crazy, right? Because you have to deliver on your work, and you have to take care of the house, and there is the child who is studying. (Brown woman, thirty-two years old, Sapopemba, São Paulo, SP)

The increase in remote working further blurred the division between the contexts of "work" and "home." Domestic tasks that were usually perceived as a break, or as a way to be distracted and relaxed from formal work, became a burden, whereas paid work started to creep beyond formal working hours:

> At home, I couldn't do the same time I did at work. I extended it, because there were days when I couldn't fulfil my workload within my working hours, because of my housework, because I had to cook, I had to take care of the house, I had to take care of it all. We work twice as hard at home, taking care of the house, taking care of remote work. (white woman, thirty-nine years old, Sapopemba, São Paulo, SP)

> I had a job outside the house, you know, I went, I left the house, but I also had a job at home, the same job I do today, only as I went out, I saw other people, there

> were other adult interactions, right? So the work was much easier. Sometimes I got home, it was a time to really relax, to, you know, put your feet up. Sometimes, there was something to do and such, but we would do it quickly, and we would have fun, the house was that moment of distraction. And now, it's really a job, because you're here all the time, you don't have anywhere else to go, there's work all the time, because at home the work never ends, you know. (Brown woman, thirty-two years old, Cabana do Pai Tomás, Belo Horizonte, MG)

The feeling of nonstop work reported by interviewees was a common experience during the pandemic that particularly impacted women (Antunes 2020). Working from home resulted in increased individualization of work and distance from union organizations, resulting in greater social isolation and a trend toward the elimination of worker rights, as well as lack of separation between the formal working time and personal time (Antunes 2020).

Unemployment, Informal Work, and Precarity

Women described a perceived increase in precarious and informal work during the pandemic:

> I see another wound in the job market with this issue of the CLT [Consolidation of Labor Laws] of working hours. . . . Today I see my sister working in a space that was supposed to be through the CLT system, and it's a contract; that is, when this contract ends, she leaves and she won't have any guaranteed rights, guarantee salary, vacation days, anything. (Black woman, forty-three years old, Sapopemba, São Paulo, SP)

The gig economy, or as it is usually referred to in Brazil, the "uberization" of work, was one of the main ways workers coped with the economic crises during the pandemic. Sewing masks was one of the most common activities women got involved in to maintain income during the beginning of the pandemic, as there was a widespread shortage:

> One of the things that helped us a lot was . . . the masks, which my mother was making. At the beginning, there was a good return, we managed to get by with what we were getting from the masks and the emergency aid. (Black woman, twenty-six years old, Sapopemba, São Paulo, SP)

Brazilian women had to create work for themselves, as the only possible option in a context of total neglect by the government:

> I think people had to sort of find a way for themselves to make an income. Invent things to do at home, to sell online. So, at my house, where I lived with my mother, she had to find a way to survive, she opened a car wash, in front of the house. She

> also tried to open a wine cellar. (Black woman, twenty-three years old, Sapopemba, São Paulo, SP)

Labor changes were also observed among those with formal jobs, especially in the care sector, which was in high demand during the pandemic, when caregivers were required to work extensive hours without the right to have time off.

> I work as a caregiver, right? I returned [from vacation] now on the 16th of May, and yes, there were changes. When I returned, I learned that I cannot have my monthly time off; if I work 12 hours, I usually get 36 hours off, and all people who work 12 by 36 are entitled to a monthly time off, and my time off has been cut. So, I won't be entitled until further notice, which I don't know when it will be. So, I think it was a very drastic change, because if you work every other day, you work 12 hours a day, there comes a time at the end of the month when you're super tired. (Brown woman, sixty-four years old, Sapopemba, São Paulo, SP)

Many of those workers who experienced precarity were Black women, family providers, and those who worked in care-associated roles, who were unable to socially isolate due to the dual challenges of the care function and the need to earn a living, both of which posed a direct risk of COVID-19 infection.

> When we look at the death rates, since when it started, right, with the maids who were circulating there in the house of the "cool" ones, are the Black women who need to go to work, the majority who are underemployed, who live in very precarious conditions, these are the ones that to guarantee a livelihood have circulate more. (Black woman, forty-three years old, Sapopemba, São Paulo, SP)

Work and Well-Being

The COVID-19 crisis also caused mental distress, with increasing cases of anxiety, depression, and stress (Miranda et al. 2020). Significant research (FIOCRUZ 2020) has shown the gendered nature of this mental health challenge, with women being more affected than men, mainly due to the structural inequalities they suffer.

> Women, mothers of families, I believe we're the most affected by this pandemic. Because before, the kids were at school, and they [the women] went out looking for work. And, today, there is neither one nor the other: neither the kids are in school, nor can they go out looking for work, you know? And it turns out that this leaves the person a little more "down," without hope, thinking that this difficult situation will last for the rest of their lives. (Brown woman, twenty-five years old, Cabana do Pai Tomás, Belo Horizonte, MG)

This vignette depicts a woman, a mother, who believes that she and other women in the same condition as her are the most affected by the pandemic, as she now feels "without hope," as if the pandemic would "last for the rest of her life." This hopelessness comes as women are often left with the sole responsibility of caring for their households and families. Therefore, in a situation where employment is not guaranteed, they are left in a position where they have to make sacrifices: stop going out looking for work and take care of their kids, who were staying at home (as the interviewee highlighted). Respondents expressed how their stress and anxiety was directly related to paid and unpaid work:

> For me it was really difficult, it was a shock, right, because you start to think how you, with two small children, are going to get a job in the middle of a pandemic. I was desperate. (Black woman, thirty-three years old, Sapopemba, São Paulo, SP)

The quote above represents what several women shared in the interviews: mental distress was caused by a lack of ability to find work while being responsible to financially support their families during the pandemic, while simultaneously being overloaded with household and care labor. Women's mental distress during the pandemic was also related to food insecurity, as they were often the ones responsible for preparing food for their families:

> Not having food at home, it is much harder for the woman than for the man. Because she is the one who is making food for her family. That was up to us, so I think we suffer a lot more. (Indigenous woman, fifty-eight years old, Cabana do Pai Tomás, Belo Horizonte, MG)

Women were also affected by their husband's unemployment, which in turn, was identified as a cause of domestic violence:

> Perhaps the husband is unemployed, and the wife is at home, both staying indoors, the fights are more constant. And I think that if there is a difference between men and women, it is that women suffer more, they end up enduring more, you know? And then there's violence. (Brown woman, sixty-four years old, Sapopemba, São Paulo, SP)

In face of these challenges, women stressed the need for psychological support tailored to their needs:

> I think there should be more psychological support. For women, you know? When the woman is more overloaded, the psychological more affected, I think she should have support. (Brown woman, fifty years old, Cabana do Pai Tomás, Belo Horizonte, MG)

Assessment of Government Policies Related to Work

> There are mothers who have lost their jobs and have not been able to recover until today. . . . So, what the government could have done is to maintain the income of these people, right, since unfortunately a pandemic came, unfortunately many people died because of it, and the population had to stay at home, it had to provide conditions for these people to stay home and not starve. (Brown woman, twenty-five years old, Cabana do Pai Tomás, Belo Horizonte, MG)

The interviewees expressed their dissatisfaction with the lack of social support from the government for people who became unemployed during the pandemic, especially for mothers, as the reflection above shows the plight of the domestic workers, who were among the most vulnerable workers during the pandemic.

> I think the government had to give people a structure, because they can't stop working, otherwise, they die of hunger at home . . . the person who has a better financial structure can afford to stay at home, or can afford to take many jobs, to do home office. Now, people, a cleaning lady, for example, can she stop working? (white woman, twenty-seven years old, Cabana do Pai Tomás, Belo Horizonte, MG)

In face of the government response gap regarding the downstream effects related to unemployment during the pandemic, women emphasized the central role of the third sector (social organizations and volunteers) in fulfilling what should have been done by public institutions in terms of giving social support to communities:

> I don't even hear about the state government, because I don't even know what it does. Now, in the municipality there are a lot of NGOs, a lot of people who are not from the government that help the people. (white woman, twenty-seven years old, Cabana do Pai Tomás, Belo Horizonte, MG)

Discussion

The COVID-19 pandemic has caused much harm, suffering, and death, besides exposing and heightening inequalities worldwide. In Brazil and other middle-income countries, the impact has been greatest among equity-deserving communities. In this context, inequalities intensified, with Black and low-income women particularly experiencing negative disruptions and changes to their working arrangements. In a country marked by diverse inequalities like Brazil, inadequate public policies to minimize the damage caused by the pandemic, layered on top of the need to physically distance for safety, led women to be overloaded with unpaid work and out of paid work.

Intersectional analysis is necessary to have a nuanced understanding of the various vulnerabilities that affect women and how these intersections can contribute to greater engagement (and advocacy) with transnational feminists. Our data show that gender inequities did not affect women at similar intensities and frequencies, and it is impossible to separate our analysis between race, class, and gender, given that they are experienced simultaneously by women. Experiences of both increased unpaid care and paid work during the pandemic were mediated by racial and income inequities alongside gender inequities. Thus, intersectionality provides theoretical-methodological instrumentality to the inseparability of racism, capitalism, and cis-heteropatriarchy in order to deepen the analysis of women's experiences during the COVID-19 pandemic.

Many women, especially Black women, lost formal employment and had to resort to informal and precarious work without social provision or access to assistance benefits (Costa, Barbosa, and Hecksher 2021). Informal work is often presented as an alternative way to achieve financial security when, in reality, workers' expectations and needs are rarely fulfilled; on the contrary, informal work places the worker in a situation of social vulnerability (Lira 2012), especially in the context of the pandemic. Informal workers are praised as inventive microentrepreneurs in a neoliberal discourse of meritocracy in the Brazilian context of weakening and precarious employment relationships and fundamental labor rights, a phenomenon known as the privilege of servitude (Antunes 2020).

Women's unemployment, which worsened during the pandemic, was heightened by several factors such as those highlighted in the interviews: gender inequalities in household and care labor, increased demand for care for children and for elderly and sick relatives, mental distress, and lack of social support from the government. For those who continued working, there were challenges related to the lack of boundaries between work and home, intensification of working hours, instability of employment ties and reduction of labor rights. The government's responses to these and the downstream effects of COVID-19 were insufficient and further inflamed by the strategy to intentionally spread the virus (Ventura, Aith, and Reis 2021).

Note

1. "Brown" is a term used by the Brazilian Institute of Geography and Statistics (IBGE, or Instituto Brasileiro de Geografia e Estatística in Portuguese) to classify one of the five groups of "race or color" that make up the Brazilian population. The IBGE is responsible for the Brazilian census, and its manual defines "brown" as the term used to characterize those with mixed skin colors (Petruccelli and Saboia 2013).

References

Abramo, Laís, and María Elena Valenzuela. 2016. "Tempo de trabalho remunerado e não remunerado na América Latina: uma repartição desigual." In *Gênero e Trabalho no Brasil e na França: Perspectivas interseccionais*, edited by Alice Rangel de Paiva Abreu and Helena Hirata, 113–124. São Paulo: Boitempo.

Akotirene, Carla. 2020. *Interseccionalidade*. São Paulo: Editora Jandaíra.

Antunes, Ricardo. 2020. *O privilégio da servidão: O novo proletariado de serviços na era digital*, 2nd ed. São Paulo: Boitempo.

Batista, Amanda, Bianca Antunes, Guilherme Faveret, Igor Peres, Janaina Marchesi, João Pedro Cunha, Leila Dantas, et al. 2020. Nota Técnica 11: Análise socioeconômica da taxa de letalidade da COVID-19 no Brasil. NOIS (Núcleo de Operações e Inteligência em Saúde). https://ponte.org/wp-content/uploads/2020/05/NT11-An%C3%A1lise-descritiva-dos-casos-de-COVID-19.pdf.

Blanc, Nathalie, Sandra Laugier, and Pascale Molinier. 2020. "O preço do invisível: As mulheres na pandemia." *Dilemas: Revista de Estudos de Conflito e Controle Social:* 1–13. https://www.reflexpandemia.org/texto-88.

Brazil Ministry of Health. 2022. "Boletim Epidemiológico N° 118—Boletim COE Coronavírus." [Epidemiological Bulletin No. 118—COE Coronavirus Bulletin]. https://www.gov.br/saude/pt-br/centrais-de-conteudo/publicacoes/boletins/epidemiologicos/covid-19/2022/boletim-epidemiologico-no-118-boletim-coe-coronavirus.pdf.

BRIDJE Institute. 2021. "Entenda tudo sobre o Programa Emergencial de Manutenção do Emprego e da Renda." Portal Politize. https://www.politize.com.br/programa-emergencial-de-manutencao-do-emprego-e-renda/.

Chancel, Lucas, Thomas Piketty, Emmanuel Saez, and Gabriel Zucman. "World Inequality Report 2022." World Inequality Lab. https://wir2022.wid.world/www-site/uploads/2022/03/0098-21_WIL_RIM_RAPPORT_A4.pdf.

DIEESE. 2022. "Economia patina, com escolhas do governo, resquícios da pandemia e crise internacional, e trabalhadores pagam a conta." https://www.dieese.org.br/boletimespecial/2022/1deMaio.html.

FIOCRUZ (Fundaçâo Oswaldo Cruz). 2020. "Saúde mental e atenção psicossocial na Pandemia COVID-19—Recomendações Gerais." FIOCRUZ. https://www.fiocruzbrasilia.fiocruz.br/wp-content/uploads/2020/04/Saúde-Mental-e-Atenção-Psicossocial-na-Pandemia-Covid-19-recomendações-gerais.pdf.

Fundo Brasil. 2022. Mapeamento do Trabalho Informal no Brasil. Fundo Brasil. https://www.fundobrasil.org.br/wp-content/uploads/2023/01/mapeamento-trabalho-informal-corte1-1.pdf.

Gênero e Número. 2020a. "'Nossa lei é a que vale': Com mais de 70% das domésticas na informalidade, condições de empregadores prevalecem sobre a PEC." https://www.generonumero.media/nossa-lei-e-que-vale-com-mais-de-70-das-domesticas-na-informalidade-condicoes-de-empregadores-prevalecem-sobre-pec/.

Gênero e Número. 2020b. "Trabalhadoras informais temem não ter como alimentar os filhos em crise do coronavírus." https://www.generonumero.media/trabalhadoras-informais-temem-nao-ter-como-alimentar-os-filhos-em-crise-do-coronavirus/.

Guimarães, Nadya Araújo, and Helena Sumiko Hirata. 2020. *O gênero do cuidado: desigualdades, significações e identidades*. São Paulo: Ateliê Editorial.

Hogan, Vijaya K., Edna M. de Araujo, Kia L. Caldwell, Sarah N. Gonzalez-Nahm, and Kristin Z. Black. 2018. "'We Black Women Have to Kill a Lion Everyday': An Intersectional Analysis of Racism and Social Determinants of Health in Brazil." *Social Science and Medicine* 199: 96–105. https://doi.org/10.1016/j.socscimed.2017.07.008.

Lira, Izabel Cristina Dias. 2012. "Trabalho informal como alternativa ao desemprego: desmistificando a informalidade." In *Políticas públicas de trabalho e renda no Brasil contemporâneo*, 3rd ed., edited by Maria Ozanira da Silva and Maria Carmelita Yazbek, 169–208. São Paulo: Cortez.

Miranda, Tainara Sales, Gustavo Fonseca Genelhu Soares, Bruna Elblink Araujo, Gabriel Henrique Alves Fagundes, Hendel Lucas Pereira do Amaral, Hian Campos Soares, Kamila Santos Tavares, et al. 2020. "Incidência dos casos de transtornos mentais durante a pandemia da COVID-19." *Revista Eletrônica Acervo Científico* 17: e4873. https://doi.org/10.25248/reac.e4873.2020.

Nieto, Mercedes Pedrero. 2014. "Importancia del trabajo no remunerado: su medición y valoración mediante las encuestas de uso del tiempo." In *Uso del tiempo y trabajo no remunerado en México*, edited by Brigida Garcia and Edith Pacheco. Mexico City: Centro de Estudios Demográficos, Urbanos y Ambientales.

PENSSAN Network. 2022. "II Vigisan: National Survey on Food Insecurity in the Context of COVID-19 Pandemic in Brazil." https://olheparaafome.com.br/wp-content/uploads/2022/09/OLHESumExecutivoINGLES-Diagramacao-v2-R01-02-09-20224212.pdf.

Petruccelli, José Luis, and Ana Lucia Saboia, eds. 2013. *Características Étnico-raciais da População. Classificações e Identidades*. Rio de Janeiro: Instituto Brasileiro de Geografia e Estatística (IBGE).

Prates, Ian, Marcia Lima, Wesley M. Oliveira, Evandro L. Alves, Alexandre Nogueira, and Maria L. Duarte. 2021. "Nota Técnica No. 34: Desigualdades raciais e de gênero aumentam a mortalidade por COVID-19, mesmo dentro da mesma ocupação." *Rede de Pesquisa Solidária, Boletim* 34. https://redepesquisasolidaria.org/wp-content/uploads/2021/09/boletimpps-34-20set2021-1.pdf.

Ramos, Edith Maria Barbosa, Paulo Roberto Barbosa Ramos, and Laísse Lima Silva Costa. 2020. "Pandemia e federalismo: reflexões sobre as decisões do Supremo Tribunal Federal na apreciação de conflitos de competência entre os entes federativos no enfrentamento à COVID-19." *Revista Ciências Jurídicas e Sociais* 1 (1): 46–61.

Ribas, Rafaela. 2021. "Mulheres dedicam quase o dobro do tempo do que homens à tarefa do lar." O Globo, March 4. https://oglobo.globo.com/economia/celina/noticia/2021/03/mulheres-dedicam-quase-dobro-do-tempo-do-que-homens-tarefas-do-lar-24908717.ghtml.

Teixeira, Marilane. 2020. "Sem Parar: O trabalho e a vida das mulheres na pandemia." *Sempreviva Organização Feminista.* https://mulheresnapandemia.sof.org.br/efeitos-pandemia-mulheres-trabalhadoras/.

Ventura, Deisy, Fernando Aith, and Rossana Reis. 2021. "Crimes against Humanity in Brazil's COVID-19 Response: A Lesson to Us All." *BMJ* 375: n2625. https://doi.org/10.1136/bmj.n2625.

Wenham, Clare, Michelle Fernandez, Marcela Garcia Corrêa, Gabriela Lotta, Brunah Schall, Mariela Campos Rocha, and Denise Nacif Pimenta. 2022. "Gender and Race on the Frontline: Experiences of Health Workers in Brazil during the COVID-19 Pandemic." *Social Politics: International Studies in Gender, State & Society* 29 (4): 1144–1167.

World Bank. 2018. "Population Living in Slums (% of Urban Population)—Brazil." https://data.worldbank.org/indicator/EN.POP.SLUM.UR.ZS?locations=BR.

4 "A Double-Edged Sword": Lived Experiences of Recent Immigrant Women in British Columbia, Canada, during COVID-19

Alice Mũrage and Julia Smith

Introduction

The first case of COVID-19 was detected in British Columbia (BC), Canada, on January 28, 2020, with case numbers continuing to rise into April 2020 and then decline due to a province-wide lockdown that restricted individual interaction. Following this initial wave, BC saw subsequent waves of infection rise and fall over the next two years and beyond. While men were overrepresented in COVID-19-related hospitalization and mortality (53 percent compared to 47 percent), women were overrepresented in the number of cases overall, largely due to their frontline role in the health services (54 percent compared to 46 percent) (Government of Canada 2022a). While race-disaggregated data are limited in Canada, the available data indicate that racialized populations disproportionately died from COVID-19; this has been associated with socioeconomic marginalization related to employment, income, and housing opportunities (Gupta and Aitken 2022). Further, racialized immigrants were overrepresented in frontline and service sectors with greater risk of exposure to COVID-19 (Statistics Canada 2020).

In addition to the primary health effects of the pandemic, public health measures put in place from March 2020—such as closures of childcare centers, schools, education institutions, and businesses—contributed to secondary socioeconomic effects. Losses in employment and income, increases in gender-based violence, and negative mental health outcomes disproportionately impacted women, racialized groups, and immigrants (Statistics Canada 2020; Shrma et al. 2022; Smith et al. 2022). For instance, the highest employment losses in the first wave of the pandemic were reported among recently immigrated women, 20 percent of whom lost jobs from March 2020 to

April 2020 (Hou, Picot, and Zhang 2020). While the government responded to widespread income losses by providing financial aid to individuals, the eligibility criteria limited accessibility (Smith et al. 2022).

In this chapter, we highlight the experiences of racialized recent immigrant women during the COVID-19 pandemic in BC, Canada, illustrating how their social location—characterized by social and economic marginalization associated with their identity as women (gender), their race or ethnicity, and their status as recent immigrants—determined their vulnerability to the secondary effects of the pandemic and how they demonstrated resilience within this context. In doing so we draw on the foundational intersectional scholarship of African American feminists (Crenshaw 1989) as well as recent applications of this scholarship to critical health studies (Bowleg 2023). As others have written, gender inequalities underlie migratory processes, and the experience of migration is shaped by multiple social locations (Parreñas 2009). In line with the other chapters in this volume, we emphasize how broader structural inequities shape women's experiences of a health crisis, particularly highlighting those that intersect with race and immigration status. We particularly focus on how the COVID-19 pandemic illuminated the relationship between inequities in paid work and unpaid care work and the resultant impacts on women's well-being.

We recognize that these outcomes are shaped by prepandemic structural inequities. Intersectionality scholars rightly call for an interrogation of context, as it is systems and structures, not intersecting identities in and of themselves, that shape societal inequities. Similarly, Park (2011), writing about the experiences of women of Asian descent, emphasizes the importance of understanding how immigrant and racialized women are positioned within Canada's globalized economy and politics of settler nationalism. In Canada, historically produced, structural inequities, such as a wage gap of 16 percent, continue to limit women's income and food security. Gender norms designate women in Canada as primary caregivers, with women doing on average two to three times more unpaid care work than men, including childcare, eldercare, and housework (Moyster and Burlock 2018). Racialized women are particularly affected by structural and interpersonal racism, which contributes to socioeconomic marginalization and mental unwellness (Williams et al. 2022). Prior to the pandemic, recent immigrant women were overrepresented among those living below the poverty line in Canada and in precarious employment. Their employment options continue to be limited by language barriers, lack of recognition of prior academic or professional qualifications, and racism. While both the federal and BC provincial governments have committed to integrating gender-based analysis into policy responses, including the COVID-19 response, Cameron and Tedds (2020) note that the government has been complicit in the systems that construct the inequities gender-based analysis seeks to rectify. A civil society report card on the BC government found that women and gender-diverse individuals from groups made the most vulnerable are most often excluded from the benefits of supposedly equity-based policies (Sproule and Prochuk 2020).

Methods

We draw from lived experiences of racialized recent immigrant women in BC, Canada, as narrated through twenty semistructured interviews. We define "recent immigrant" as anyone who immigrated to Canada ten or fewer years before the pandemic, and "racialized" as anyone who does not identify as white or Caucasian. The data presented in this chapter were collected in two parts: eight interviews during the initial lockdown (May to June 2020) and twelve interviews between September and December 2021. This enabled an analysis of both the immediate and ongoing effects on this group of women. Most participants were parents, and they ranged in age from eighteen to fifty. They represented a variety of ethnicities, coming from Asia, Africa, Latin America, and the Middle East. When necessary, interpretation services were provided to interviewees. We also conducted interviews with six key informants from civil society organizations that advocate for women's and immigrant rights to gain a deeper understanding of the broader context. Interview transcripts were analyzed using reflexive thematic analysis, wherein both authors familiarized themselves with the data and then coconstructed codes and then themes (Braun et al. 2019).

Results

Career Interruptions and Economic Impacts

Prior to COVID-19, immigrant women already experienced structural and social barriers that hindered their participation in the Canadian labor market. Among the women we interviewed, language barriers and lack of recognition of foreign credentials and work experience were particularly significant in limiting their ability to pursue work that aligned with their qualifications and interests. Women described moving to Canada as being "born again" and having to "start from zero" in terms of learning a new language and pursuing Canadian credentials and work experience.

> As a new immigrant in Canada, it's not—I think it's not easy. Because all—in Shanghai we have a comfortable life. We all did senior office jobs. But now if you came to here, you just learn people, the English language; and all that you did before have become zero. So maybe to a newcomer it's not easy. . . . I have the master's degree in my country. But now I have to start from zero. (immigrant from China, unpartnered, one child)

The pandemic created new impediments to the process of starting over, disrupting plans to take language classes and build careers.

> I have masters [degree] and license in my country, I don't want here just be like a food worker. I want to improve. I want to go to the school to learn English. I was applying for Pathway [a health education program in a local college]. I wanted to take my English 12 [minimum English competence level for entry to some colleges] because I wanted to take a program. But right now, [the college] is not working, any college is not working because of COVID-19. (immigrant from Iran, partnered, two children)

Even when such classes were transitioned to online learning, many women expressed difficulty learning a language through virtual interactions, and many did not have the necessary technology to participate.

The COVID-19 pandemic had a significant impact on the Canadian economy across industries. This impact was particularly pronounced following the first wave of the pandemic and subsequent public health measures, which resulted in business and in-person service closures starting in March 2020. However, impacts on paid work were differential. For instance, immigrant workers lost more work hours than Canadian-born workers, immigrant women lost more hours than immigrant men, and racialized immigrants lost more hours than white immigrants (Shrma, Smith, and Mũrage, 2022). These trends reflect the overrepresentation of immigrants and women in precarious employment and in the low-paying sectors most impacted by pandemic shutdowns, such as the accommodation, food service, and tourism sectors. Reflecting these trends, most respondents had also lost income or employment since the start of the pandemic due to business closures and reduced business capacities. As many were in precarious employment positions before the pandemic, those who remained employed were made more precarious as the number of hours available for work were dependent on market demands. Restaurant workers, for instance, reported unpredictable working hours and income, where one could earn between CAD (Canadian dollars) 1,500 and CAD 3,000 per month depending on assigned hours. Income earnings were notably more variable compared to pre-COVID incomes, which were more reliable. One woman noted that her income dropped to below CAD 500 per month.

> instead of working seven days she is now working only two days and one of those days is just on call. . . . And when they told them to return back to work for these two days [during the pandemic], it was, like, the whole day [earning] less than 150 dollars a day. Like, the two checks for the month, less than 500 dollars. (as interpreted; immigrant from Egypt, unpartnered, no children)

Canada's initial pandemic response aimed to mitigate financial hardship caused by lost income through financial relief initiatives, the largest of which was the Canada Emergency Response Benefit (CERB): This provided 2,000 Canadian Dollars (CAD) per month to those who had lost income due to the COVID-19 pandemic and met the eligibility criteria of having earned more than CAD 5,000 of taxable income in the previous year (Government of Canada 2022b). Those respondents who accessed CERB noted that it provided welcome relief.

> In Canada I really, really appreciate government, they help the people, you know. We are newcomers here, if government didn't help us, didn't care for us, we couldn't withstand this time. How could we pay for our house, and right now we pay for our house CAD 2,200. So, they care about people. (immigrant from Iran, partnered, two children)

Following the initial months of the pandemic, CERB was transitioned to the Canada Recovery Benefit in October 2020, which provided financial relief for another fifty-two weeks and for which many respondents qualified due to continued unemployment or reduced hours. However, several respondents did not fully access the available financial supports due to a desire to be self-reliant and present a good example for their children. One noted,

> I [don't] want my son to know your mum just get the government to fund to live in Canada. So I stopped it. I think—I just thought to myself I can study harder. I can work harder. (immigrant from China, unpartnered, one child)

Many women expressed that it was work, not support, that they needed: "I'm not into it [CERB] because I just want to earn and, like by my own" (immigrant from Pakistan, unpartnered, no children).

Similarly, an interpreter communicated for a recently arrived woman,

> She mentioned that she prefers to work more than staying at home and receiving benefits from the government. She applied for them when she really, really needed that, to survive. But otherwise, she usually, like, preferred to work and earn money. (immigrant from Egypt, unpartnered, no children)

Despite the preference for employment opportunities, respondents highlighted struggles returning to the labor market after public health measures were lifted and businesses began to reopen their doors. In 2020, recent immigrant women recorded lower rates of transition from unemployment to employment at the start of partial recovery (Hou, Picot, and Zhang 2020); this could partly be explained by the employment options open to this demographic.

As immigration offices closed during the initial months of the pandemic, resulting in a backlog when services reopened, many respondents also experienced delays in their settlement process, which impacted their ability to work.

> I understand that because of the COVID-19, everything got delay and my application is being affected. . . . I submitted my PR [permanent residence] application on May 29th. Immigration received on May 29th and we do all the documents and everything and then the medical examination. And then the last communication was on February 10th, last communication from immigration that we all passed the medical exam, so that's it. So, the note there is they are now for final decision. So, I was expecting the March or April I will receive my PR card or my PR approval. But because of COVID, it got delayed. (immigrant from the Philippines, partner and two children in the Philippines)

Another woman noted that her work permit had expired, and while she had applied for an extension months ago, she had yet to receive a reply. A woman who had recently arrived in Canada had not yet received a work permit, and thus could not take on employment and was not eligible for financial relief programs because she had not worked in Canada previously.

Barriers to employment (and to accessing support benefits) contributed to housing insecurity and fear of homelessness, particularly in the context of an affordability crisis in BC, where both housing and food costs increased throughout the pandemic. Several women had to move to different apartments during the pandemic, reporting significant increases in rental expenses; one noted a 45 percent increase in her rent. The combination of increased living costs and decreased or more precarious income caused high levels of stress and anxiety.

Coping with Unpaid Care Burdens

When the pandemic and subsequent public health measures resulted in closures of childcare centers, schools, and community resources, women disproportionately carried the additional care burden. For instance, in Canada in 2020, 64 percent of women reported providing most homeschooling support, compared to 19 percent of men (Leclerc 2020). Such gender roles shaped the experiences of recent immigrant women, who also faced unique burdens due to their newcomer status in Canada.

In Canada, childcare offered by relatives is the second most used childcare arrangement (Findlay 2019); this is not an option available to many newcomers. Over half of the women interviewed had no extended family in Canada. While a majority had a nuclear family, with some immigrating through spousal sponsorship, others were single parents, which further isolated them socially and disadvantaged them economically. Support networks that had been fostered with friends and neighbors were restricted by pandemic policies around physical distancing. One single mother described how she had to give up her job when she could no longer rely on neighbors to care for her child. Another quit her part-time job in the service industry out of recognition that childcare through neighbors (which allowed her to pursue employment) increased her child's risk of infection.

> I went through a lot. I used to work and then after I said, no, I can't sacrifice my son because there is not anyone who will take care of him. I always gave him to neighbors. They really help me [but] it's not [safe] for my child to be babysat with more people. Like today's this one, today's this one; so it's really affected me mentally, emotionally. (immigrant from the Democratic Republic of the Congo, unpartnered, one child)

Lack of childcare inhibited mothers' ability to access necessities during the initial lockdown when long lines and supply chain disruptions made shopping time-consuming. One mother explained,

> At that moment everybody was doing grocery shopping and I didn't have stuff at home because I used to buy my groceries per week, and that moment I asked my neighbor, "Can you look after my son, I need to go for milk and eggs and I don't want to bring my son there" and she said, "Sorry, I can't because you are working and I don't know if you were exposed to the virus." . . . I can't be three hours in the line when sometimes—because we get there, there was no meat, no eggs, no milk—and so you may see the long line to get inside the store and nothing. (immigrant from Mexico, unpartnered one child)

Many mothers had previously coped with low incomes by shopping around for the most affordable products at multiple shops. Such strategies became impossible during the pandemic.

Single mothers without social support networks were forced to take their children shopping at a time when this was discouraged through public health advisories. This shopping experience was described as stressful because of associated social stigma. One mother noted feeling "like a bad mom" and another described experiencing "mom guilt." One respondent reported that a cashier chastised her for bring her son to the grocery store:

> Grocery shopping and supply shopping has been a challenge again because they really encourage you not to go with your child, but when you're a single mom what are you going to do? Leave the kid home? So that has definitely been a challenge. I did take her a few times to the local Safeway store and I had very judgy eyes. (immigrant from Japan, unpartnered, one child)

Additionally, it was challenging to manage children's patience where cashier queues, as respondents noted, could be "1–2 kilometers long" with "no special time or line for people with little kids." One mother shared how on some occasions she was forced to go back home without needed necessities because of such queues. Anxiety over COVID-19 infections was heightened during shopping where children "touched everything" and access to PPE was limited. One responded shared, "We couldn't find masks; we couldn't find hand sanitizer for maybe one and half months" (immigrant from Iran, partnered, two children).

Some women also shared that they could not find nutritious food for their children. One single mother named this as her biggest fear at the time:

> I wasn't scared about getting sick, but my fear was I don't have food for my son in the fridge. That was my biggest fear because I know I have money in my bank account, but there is nothing in the store. (immigrant from Mexico, unpartnered, one child)

Both federal and provincial governments provided extra funding to community-based organizations that provided necessities to immigrants, and many women described the benefits of these programs. A number had accessed food banks or similar supports.

> There is [a community organization] close to my home, they start to give us some groceries, and then they send me a lot because they start to send me the eggs and the milk and they give me a little bit of meat, and then that helped me a lot because then I don't need to go to the store with my son. So that was really good. (immigrant from Mexico, unpartnered, one child)

One woman explained that at first, she was scared to go to the food bank, as she feared it would affect her permanent residence application, but then was relieved when a nonprofit supporting domestic workers brought the food to her house and did not take any contact information.

Even after formal childcare facilities reopened to the public in July 2020 and employment opportunities began to recover, formal childcare was inaccessible to many immigrant women due to limited availability and prohibitive costs. A pre-COVID-19 study found that childcare fees in most cities were unaffordable, and another noted that 44 percent of non-school-aged children lived in "childcare deserts" where there are not enough childcare spaces available to meet needs (Macdonald 2018; Macdonald and Friendly 2020). BC in particular has a legacy of high fees and few spaces. A 2018 survey found that 46.5 percent of BC families with children under five had difficulty accessing childcare (Edwards 2020). Precarious, low-wage work combined with economic loss during lockdown meant most respondents could not afford childcare fees even if they could find childcare.

> Economically I just felt like you know having to pay CAD 2,000 a month I just really couldn't afford it especially because my contract was cancelled. So, I really made that decision because I thought you know it's better for him not to be in daycare [due to fear of infection] and honestly, I really can't afford it. (immigrant from Columbia, unpartnered, one child)

The same single mother similarly noted she lost both her job and childcare during the initial months of the pandemic and subsequently found it challenging to find a new job:

> You know, it's challenging for a single mom to be able to go back to work and having to pay. It's kind of a double-edged sword because you need the daycare [to work] and yet you know if you aren't working you can't pay for daycare. So, you almost need it, but you only need it when you are going to work. (immigrant from Columbia, unpartnered, one child)

Another noted she had tried to do a phone interview for a new job, but her children kept interrupting her, prompting the interviewer to ask if she had childcare. She noted, "I didn't hear back after that" (immigrant from Afghanistan, unpartnered, two children).

During school closures, lack of equipment (such as laptops), language barriers, and unfamiliarity with the Canadian education system created unique challenges for newcomer mothers responsible for homeschooling their children.

> His teacher sent the homework and [said] I should study first by myself and then explain to my son "you should do this, you should do that" and was really difficult for me. That was a big headache for me because it's so hard . . . You know if you were good in English your problem is less, but I wasn't, I'm not good in English language and everything that we learned in school is different than here, for example about division, about multiples. I can't—I know how I should multiply two number but I can't explain to him. And the way here, the way is different with that I taught in my country. (immigrant from Iran, partnered, two children)

Another noted how her child had to use her phone to engage in online classes and yet another noted that closure of public libraries meant her daughter did not have access to books.

> Only one thing is very hard for me is the pandemic, the school is closed. The school closing is for me very, very hard. I need to teach the kids online. It's very hard. I'm almost crazy. (immigrant from China, partnered, two children)

Mental Wellness and Resilience

The above-described effects on paid and unpaid labor, and consequent challenges with accessing necessities, generated stress, anxiety and depression. While mental health deteriorated across the Canadian population during the first year of the pandemic, studies have found that both women and immigrants were particularly affected (Evra and Mongrain 2020). The women included in this study faced sources of anxiety related to both their context in Canada and concern for those in their country of origin. This dual-country experience added an additional layer of stress. A woman from Iran explained, "And I'm worried for my family in our country because the number of people who suffered in my country were more than here" (immigrant from Iran, partnered, two children).

Another woman expressed concern about sending remittances home while laid off due to COVID-19, recognizing that the costs of living for her family in the Philippines had risen sharply.

Many also expressed severe loneliness and a sense of isolation that, while common particularly during lockdown and periods when physical distancing was required, were particularly poignant for recent immigrants who did not have extended social networks. A young woman explained,

> I feel like so lonely at home. And then so I have also roommate next to my room but I couldn't—yeah, I couldn't see her [during isolation]. And then also I'm alone so I don't have any family here. (immigrant from Japan, unpartnered, no children)

Several commented on the challenge of adapting to a new culture in such an exceptional situation.

> It's because when you come here as an immigrant, we don't have the community and networking, like you don't know anyone. I guess some of us they're just lonely; like I'm counting myself. I just have a few friends around and you don't know that many people and the culture. The culture of people getting together, like of those things, like when this COVID comes they just feel very lonely because they cannot see anyone and the online part is not something they understand. (immigrant from Iran, partnered, no children)

Some women mentioned how the closure of in-person religious gatherings compounded their sense of isolation and prevented them from accessing a support network they counted on. As English as a second language classes moved online, this previous avenue for meeting new people was also reduced.

> So, the mosques and churches are closed. Schools are not in person. Like, they are teaching us virtually. And I have been in school for one year and I don't know who were my class fellows, and I haven't seen anyone. Not even my teachers . . . If you're talking to someone, you will get to know many things about their culture, their—you can say it's inner peace, talk with someone, what I feel. But I missed that for one year. (immigrant from Pakistan, unpartnered, no children)

Lack of social and family support heightened anxiety around COVID-19 infection. A single mother explained,

> My fear is that, like, if I get sick, who is going to look after my son—because I don't have no one . . . There is no one else if I get sick. I don't want to think about it. (immigrant from Afghanistan, partnered, two children)

Another mother explained how she restricted her children's interactions because of fear of infection: "I told them if one of them going to be sick it's very difficult for us because we don't have support here" (immigrant from Iran, partnered, two children).

A woman working as a domestic worker got COVID-19 from the family she provided childcare services to and had to deal with severe illness on her own.

> I was afraid to go to the hospital at the time. So when I got sick I didn't go to, I just stayed at home. I have fever but I just did the natural way because it's very hard. I'm coughing and have fever for 13 days and I cannot eat and everything. . . . So I prepared my room and everything, I packed my things so in case that I will die in the hospital, I said I wrote a letter that I said, "Send all my things to the Philippines and everything." (immigrant from the Philippines, with partner and two children in the Philippines)

Such experiences, as well as the anxiety and challenges noted above, affected respondents' mental health, with many describing themselves as depressed, unable to focus, and losing sleep. While the provincial government expanded virtual counseling and mental health services during the pandemic, none of the women we spoke to accessed these services. A service provider noted that stigma around mental health needs and lack of culturally appropriate services created barriers to access.

> Sometimes there is stigma. The moment that somebody finds out that they are in need of counseling services, then they will be labeled as people with issues. And sometimes the notion of counseling, for many cultures and communities, is not the same as our notion of counseling care in Canada. Mostly, in many communities, they would rely on family members for support as the counseling piece and sometimes it's the language barrier, or knowing about the information. Even though we pretty much use social media, word of mouth, different outreach to let people know, but not everybody is aware of the services there. (key informant interview, community service provider)

Others did not have access to the space or technology to participate in virtual counseling. Care available through private providers was inaccessible to those without medical benefits, and most of our respondents were employed in precarious, nonunionized positions without benefits. One woman had previously accessed counseling through her employment benefits, but that access ended when she was laid off during the pandemic.

Several respondents did find innovative and meaningful sources of support through peer networks that adapted to the challenges of the COVID-19 context.

> I was a part of a single mom's group. And so we usually have group meetings on Wednesdays but because of COVID that's changed. We can't meet in person anymore, so we've been meeting online through Zoom. There used to be childcare for the mums that have their kids with them. So that they're able to leave the kids with the childcare provider and have that two hours, and we can get into topics a little bit more detailed. Because of the fact that this is now you know the moms are at home, and this is happening at home, it's more like a one-hour meeting and moms usually join you know if kids are sleeping hopefully by then and—or you know they're occupied or something. (immigrant from Japan, unpartnered, one child)

Another woman described the support she received from an organization supporting domestic workers.

> I'm very thankful to them. And you know, that time too, it's very hard that you're sick and then you don't have somebody to talk with, anytime in the middle of the

> night, especially I was so really depressed that time, I just call them, very approachable, and they would just listen and then they brought me through different kinds of program, webinar program on Zoom that time for counseling. We are many among the group and every time we share, we cry, we cry together. That's the only way that we can maybe relieve ourselves from this burden. (immigrant from the Philippines, with partner and two children in the Philippines)

With limited support options, immigrant women described relying on their inner strength and determination. One woman, for example, described how she noticed isolation was affecting her children and so she decided to start a small catering business from her home to "show them how to be busy, to make good use of her time. And in order, like, not to get depressed." Others found contacting friends and family in their home countries helpful. Others shared the importance of positive self-affirmation in caring for their mental well-being. "I tell myself, just be patient. You all are healthy. Your family are healthy and just do a routine. Don't worry. Try to do some positive—to think positive and just be thankful." (immigrant from Iran, partnered, two children).

Discussion

The experiences of recent immigrant women in BC, Canada, during the COVID-19 pandemic is shaped by a combination of factors including immigration status, race, and gender. Recent immigrant women's experiences of career interruptions and economic loss was particularly shaped by their racialized and newcomer position within the BC economy. The initial COVID-19 lockdown did not just interrupt their employment; it stalled career development by delaying opportunities to learn English and develop local experience. With recent immigrant women overrepresented in precarious, low-wage employment in the sectors most impacted by physical distancing policies, this group saw the greatest drop in employment over the longest period (Hou, Picot, and Zhang 2020). While many were able to access financial relief, immigrant women recognized that such support did not provide what they needed most to build a life in Canada—meaningful work—and thus strove to be self-sufficient. They did so in a context of not only pandemic uncertainty but also rising housing and food costs and reduced access to settlement support services.

These experiences were structured by gender norms that made mothers more likely than fathers to be responsible for childcare and homeschooling when facilities closed or children had to stay home due to COVID-19 exposure or illness. With little access to family and social networks, most of the recent immigrant women who participated in this study had to face these challenges on their own, which complicated their ability to access necessities and find work. Providing homeschooling guidance to their children was particularly challenging for mothers not familiar with the education system or still learning English themselves.

These challenges, combined with isolation in Canada and concern for family far away, caused high levels of stress, anxiety, and depression. Recent immigrant women faced barriers accessing counseling to deal with these effects due to prohibitive costs, lack of technology or privacy to engage with virtual services, and lack of culturally appropriate options. They did, however, self-organize and join peer support groups, where they found coming together with women in similar situations beneficial.

Structural inequities related to immigration policies, Canadian gender norms, and ongoing racial discrimination shaped how recent immigrant women's paid and unpaid work, and therefore well-being, were affected by the COVID-19 pandemic. This double-edged sword affected women's income, opportunities, time use, and well-being—effects that recent immigrant women mitigated through self-resilience and community support. Their achievements in settlement, supporting their families, and advancing their careers were despite of, not due to, pandemic response policies that did not take into account their unique needs or the structural inequities that shape them.

Conclusion

The COVID-19 pandemic has created an opportunity to address historical, economic, political, and multifaceted determinants of recent immigrant women's well-being. The colonial history, and present, of Canada has perpetuated norms that regulate racialized immigrants to social and economic margins that reduce their access to services. The increased precarity of work on the margins, made immigrant women vulnerable to layoffs and reduce income during the pandemic. Lack of political investment in the care economy, and lack of prioritization of the needs of racialized and immigrant women, left many of these women to fend for themselves.

The precarious and low-wage work that made recent immigrant women vulnerable to economic loss during the pandemic, as experienced across the case studies in this book, can be transformed into secure, meaningful employment, including benefits that ensure access to services during times of crisis. Language and training programs can be enhanced to take into consideration childcare and technology needs. Ongoing efforts to improve childcare access can specifically consider the unique needs of recent immigrant women, as well as developing crisis response plans that prevent disruptions in services. The civil society organizations and peer support networks that are currently providing the bulk of services to recent immigrant women could be supported through additional funding. Such interventions would buttress the determination and resilience demonstrated by participants, empowering them both during the process of settling in a new country and in the event of future health crises.

References

Bowleg, Lisa. 2023. "Beyond Intersectional Identities: Ten Intersectional Structural Competencies for Critical Health Equity." In *The Routledge Companion to Intersectionalities*, edited by Jennifer C. Nash and Samantha Pinto, 101–116. Abingdon, UK: Routledge.

Crenshaw, Kimberley. 1989. "Demarginalizing the Intersection of Race and Sex: A Black Feminist Critique of Antidiscrimination Doctrine, Feminist Theory and Antiracist Politics." *University of Chicago Legal Forum* 1 (8): 139–167.

Edwards, Melissa. 2020. "Go Figure: What You May Not Know about Child Care in B.C." *BCBusiness*, November 13. https://www.bcbusiness.ca/What-you-may-not-know-about-child-care-in-BC.

Evra, Rose, and Eric Mongrain. 2020. "Mental Health Status of Canadian Immigrants during the COVID-19 Pandemic." *Statistics Canada*. https://www150.statcan.gc.ca/n1/pub/45-28-0001/2020001/article/00050-eng.htm.

Findlay, Leanne. 2019. *Early Learning and Child Care for Children Aged 0 to 5 years: A Provincial/Territorial Portrait*. Ottawa: Statistics Canada.

Government of Canada. 2022a. "COVID-19 Epidemiology Update: Summary of COVID-19 Cases, Hospitalizations and Deaths, Testing and Variants of Concern across Canada and Over Time." https://health-infobase.canada.ca/covid-19/#a3.

Government of Canada. 2022b. "Canada Emergency Response Benefit (CERB): Closed." https://www.canada.ca/en/services/benefits/ei/cerb-application.html.

Gupta, Shikha, and Nicole Aitken. 2022. "COVID-19 Mortality among Racialized Populations in Canada and Its Association with Income." Statistics Canada. https://www150.statcan.gc.ca/n1/pub/45-28-0001/2022001/article/00010-eng.htm.

Hou, Feng, Garnett Picot, and Jue Zhang. 2020. "Transitions into and out of Employment by Immigrants during the COVID-19 Lockdown and Recovery." Statistics Canada. https://www150.statcan.gc.ca/n1/pub/45-28-0001/2020001/article/00070-eng.htm.

Leclerc, Karine. 2020. "Caring for Their Children: Impacts of COVID-19 on Parents." Statistics Canada. https://www150.statcan.gc.ca/n1/pub/45-28-0001/2020001/article/00091-eng.htm.

Macdonald, David. 2018. "Child Care Deserts in Canada." Canadian Centre for Policy Alternatives. https://www.policyalternatives.ca/publications/reports/child-care-deserts-canada.

Macdonald, David, and Martha Friendly. 2017. "Time Out: Child Care Fees in Canada 2017." Canadian Centre for Policy Alternatives. https://www.policyalternatives.ca/sites/default/files/uploads/publications/National%20Office/2017/12/Time%20Out.pdf.

Park, Hijin. 2011. "Migrants, Minorities and Economies: Transnational Feminism and the Asian/Canadian Woman Subject." *Asian Journal of Women's Studies* 17 (4): 7–38. https://doi.org/10.1080/12259276.2011.11666115.

Parreñas, Rhacel S. 2009. "Inserting Feminism in Transnational Migration Studies." Migration Online: Focus on Central and Eastern Europe. https://documentation.lastradainternational.org/lsidocs/RParrenas_InsertingFeminisminTransnationalMigrationStudies.pdf.

Shrma, Lokpriy, Julia Smith, and Alice Mũrage. 2022. "COVID-19 and Employment Loss in the Accommodation and Food Services Sector: Spotlighting Economic Impacts on Women and Immigrants during the Pandemic." Gender & COVID-19 Project. https://www.genderandcovid-19.org/resources/covid-19-and-employment-loss-in-the-accommodation-and-food-services-sector/.

Smith, Julia, Alice Mũrage, Ingrid Lui, and Rosemary Morgan. 2022. "Integrating Gender-Based Analysis Plus (GBA+) into Canada's Response to COVID-19: Lived Experiences of Lockdown in British Columbia, Canada." *Social Politics: International Studies in Gender, State & Society* 29 (4): 1168–1191. https://doi.org/10.1093/sp/jxac024.

Statistics Canada. 2020. "Impacts on Immigrants and People Designated as Visible Minorities." Government of Canada. Statistics Canada. https://www150.statcan.gc.ca/n1/pub/11-631-x/2020004/s6-eng.htm.

Williams, Monnica T., Anjalika Khanna Roy, Marie-Paule MacIntyre, and Sonya Faber. 2022. "The Traumatizing Impact of Racism in Canadians of Colour." *Current Trauma Reports* 8 (2): 17–34. https://doi.org/10.1007/s40719-022-00225-5.

5 "Because I Am a Woman, the Man Thinks They Need to Protect Me": Gendered Experience of First Responders to COVID-19 in China

Connie C. R. Gan and Sara E. Davies

Introduction

The People's Republic of China (hereafter, China) was the first country to report the outbreak of the severe acute respiratory syndrome coronavirus 2 (SARS-CoV-2) virus and COVID-19 infection in humans on December 31, 2019. Between January 2020 and July 2022, there were 5,513,700 confirmed cases of COVID-19 infection, with 23,396 deaths (World Health Organization [WHO] 2022). For the first three years of the pandemic, the Chinese government pursued a "zero COVID" approach to prevent widespread COVID-19 infections. The central government created a national emergency response mandate to combat the spread of COVID-19 in Wuhan, Hubei (the city where the virus was first reported and detected), in January 2020. This mandate was replicated across other locations where the virus was detected. The three stages of national emergency response were, first, identification and quarantine of travelers from the city where infection was detected; second, the implementation of total lockdown, with public security bureaus involved in mass surveillance and population monitoring; and third, containment with continued restrictions including movement monitoring to prevent outbreaks (i.e., QR codes to enter buildings) (Gao, Tyson, and Cheng 2022).

In China, ethics, politics, and power over care decisions during an emergency are connected with and dependent on a highly centralized model of government and political authority. While the Chinese government claims to protect human rights and promote gender equity, the state has been steadily promoting cisgender and heteronormative norms and policies (Song 2021). Marriage and birth rates have plummeted dramatically in China despite the scrapping of the one-child policy in 2018 and even increasing the accepted number of children to a three-children policy in 2021(Ren 2022). While the party-state has done little to address the underlying socioeconomic factors of work and economic pressures or to create equitable parenting policies, they have built direct pressure on childbearing, especially on urban, educated women.

The authoritarian nature of the Chinese government makes it relatively easy to track legislative changes but quite difficult to track people's freely expressed attitudes, norms, and behaviors (Long 2018). Moreover, the emergency response mandate in China during COVID-19 made it even harder to track attitudes, norms, and behaviors, especially among first-responder populations. The "zero-COVID" strategy became a sensitive topic for the government and, by extension, for those associated with, or commenting on, the strategy. This is exemplified by most of the research on COVID-19 in China being centered on the biomedical response to the virus rather than the broader social impact of the contagion (Feng et al. 2022).

The impact of these national emergency response measures has given rise to gendered experiences of infection, illness, vulnerability, and recovery (Smith et al. 2021; Wenham, Smith, and Morgan 2020). Gendered experiences overlap with age, income, ethnicity, and disability. These experiences and differences interact to create differentiated risks of exposure among populations. Of the few publications on the gendered impact of COVID-19 in China, most are on women first responders, overwhelmingly healthcare workers, who are presented as emotionally stressed due to the high pressure experienced during the outbreak (Feng et al. 2022; Gan et al. 2022). It could be argued that the low volume of such publications on this topic, reporting similar findings, reveals what is acceptable to study and publish in China when it comes to the topic of gender and care during COVID-19 in China.

First responders to COVID-19, especially in Wuhan (the primary focus of this chapter), required the deployment of health professionals (both local and those brought in from other locations) and staff from the Chinese Centre for Disease Control and Prevention (CDC) to assist with the investigation of the outbreak, as well as police and civil society responders (including those from national and international agencies). In a situation where the emergency response measures led to the total lockdown of a city with a population of over 11 million people, we were interested in knowing how health emergency first responders managed the gendered impacts of the outbreak.

We were particularly interested in knowing this given the high representation of women in both the health and civil society sectors in China (Attané 2012; International Labour Organization 2017). In this chapter, we present the experiences of three groups of people who were charged with first responder duties during the first months of the COVID-19 outbreak (January to April 2020): health professionals (medical doctors), CDC investigation team members (epidemiologists and medical doctors), and community workers (logisticians and social workers). We examine how these individuals understood the gendered impact of the health emergency on their capacity to work and how they understood the gendered impact of the crisis on the effectiveness of the emergency response. While those interviewed had a range of different intersecting characteristics and identifiers, the selection of interview candidates based on their professional roles meant that interviews focused on their professional experiences rather than relating these to other intersecting factors. This was partly due to the need for protection for those speaking to us, as they feared being identified by government. This limits the scope of our intersectional analysis.

Several studies have interviewed frontline nurses and physicians who treated COVID-19 patients (Cao et al. 2020; Gao et al. 2020; Liu et al. 2020), outlining the health and social consequences of the pandemic. The interview research available on Chinese nurses' and doctors' experiences tended to depict the gendered impact of COVID-19 on healthcare worker experiences as the chance to up-skill in emergency response and lessons to be learned, in that some women healthcare workers tended to report more posttraumatic stress and anxiety than men (Gan et al. 2022). The finding that women healthcare workers were reporting more stress than men colleagues was rarely further analyzed to establish why. In our own findings, we observed that women healthcare workers (both nurses and doctors) experienced high levels of social pressure (i.e., expectation to stay at home during lockdown measures to care at home), and their needs, including personal protection equipment and accommodation in hospitals, was not well adapted (i.e., ill-fitting equipment, lack of privacy and reliable access to clean sanitary products) (Gan et al. 2022). Researchers (Sun et al. 2021) have returned to COVID-19 survivors and their family members to document their perceived changes and sentiments during these unprecedented times. However, to date, little research has showcased the gendered experience of COVID-19 first responders—healthcare workers, those charged with investigating the outbreak, and those responsible for supporting the community—during the immediate lockdown measures from January to April 2020.

This chapter presents our research and findings in three stages. First, we provide a brief background on the status of gender equality in China prior to the COVID-19 outbreak. This background is important for understanding the prevailing social norms in China prior to the outbreak, between reform-minded gender equality laws but persistent (and possibly state-encouraged) gender stereotypes. China is not unique in that its society experiences of a bifurcated reality: formal commitments to gender equality clash with informal behaviors and biases that reward gender discrimination (Chappell and Waylen 2013). These social tensions came to the fore during the first COVID-19 emergency in China from January to April 2020. In the second section of the chapter, we present how our interview sample of individuals within the healthcare worker sector, CDC investigation sector, and community sector experienced gendered impacts and observed gendered differences during the pandemic. Our interviewees reveal how persistent gender stereotypes negatively affected equitable representation and decision-making roles during the crisis. Men were overwhelmingly represented in the decision-making roles, despite women being overwhelmingly represented in first response work, especially in the health and civil society sectors. The CDC investigation sector initially prioritized the deployment of men over women as investigators due to gender stereotypes concerning care roles at home, quarantine conditions, and suitability for fieldwork. An unexpected outcome of the interviews, discussed in the third section of the chapter, is the view among the interviewees that due to the lack of diverse representation in decision-making roles responsible for responding to the emergency, important gendered differences among populations were missed, including knowledge of violence against women and the stress experienced by men first responders.

Methodology

Research has shown that equitable representation among first responders in the care sector, and in the areas of surveillance, governance, coordination, financing, and countermeasures, is vital to ensure an effective and equitable response during emergencies (Farhall, Gibson, and Vincent 2022).

Yet it remains difficult to prioritize equitable representation in emergencies despite research showing that a lack of diversity among first responders will lead to more implementation failures in the areas of emergency preparation, response, and recovery (Bishu, McCandless, and Elias 2021; Enarson 2012). It is therefore important to ask first responders about their experience of equity management and response during a crisis (Farhall et al. 2022).

Access to first responders was possible due to our adoption of the purposive sampling technique (Braun and Clarke 2013). Researchers on the team who knew at least one CDC worker, one healthcare sector worker, and one community sector worker who had responded to the Wuhan outbreak contacted those individuals via direct message using a shared social media platform. Once an agreement to an interview was established, and the interview was held, snowball sampling followed from there from December 2020 to January 2021. Those interviewed were, ultimately, a cross-section of government and nongovernment workers (ID column of table 5.1: CDC for CDC workers, HCW for healthcare workers, and CSW for community sector workers) who were first responders during the outbreak from January to April 2020. In total, we interviewed eight women and three men, and each interview lasted approximately one hour (see table 1.1 in chapter 1). At most interviews, both authors were present and interviews were conducted in Mandarin. All eleven transcripts were translated into English, and the authors discussed and agreed on suitable Mandarin-to-English translations of idioms. All those interviewed were highly educated (postgraduate degrees) and urban located, Han ethnicity individuals. All but three (one woman and two men) were married with children. Ages varied, but most (except one woman) were age twenty-five to fifty years of age. Questions were semistructured and were designed to cover the following topics: assignment of roles, responder experiences, impacts on responders, and other observations. Transcripts were thematically coded (roles, experience, impact, and other).

The sample size is small, and we acknowledge that the results of the study need to be interpreted with caution. The value of the findings is the rarity of the study: in-depth open-question interviews with professionals about their experiences and personal reflections on the gendered impacts of the initial stages of the COVID-19 pandemic on their work as well as their relationships.

Table 5.1
Demographic characteristics of the interviewees ($n = 11$)

ID	Gender	Involved in COVID-19 response in:	Profession and position	Affiliated organization location
CDC1	Female	Wuhan	Scientist	National
CDC2	Male	Guangdong	Epidemiologist	Provincial
CDC3	Female	Beijing, Wuhan, Xinjiang	Clinician, epidemiologist	National
HCW1	Female	Jiangsu	Medical doctor	City level
HCW2	Male	Jiangsu	Medical doctor	City level
HCW3	Female	Guangdong	Medical doctor	COVID-19 designated hospital
CSW1	Female	Beijing	Social program coordinator	International NGO
CSW2	Male	Beijing	Social program coordinator	International NGO
CSW3	Female	Guangdong	Social program coordinator	International NGO
CSW4	Female	Beijing	Social worker	National NGO
CSW5	Female	Guangdong	Data analyst	National NGO

Gender Equality in China during the COVID-19 Outbreak

Over the last ten years, the Chinese government has instituted a range of gender equality laws in the workplace and introduced an antidomestic-violence law. However, in practice, social attitudes to gender equality and women's empowerment have been described as less progressive (Ren 2022). The gender stereotype of the man as the head of the household is pervasive in Chinese society, with high expectations that men must be the primary income earners (Qing 2020). Women spend more than twice as much time on housework as men and spend far more time on unpaid work than men on average. The average time spent on housework is two hours and six minutes for women versus forty-five minutes for men per day; in 2018, women in rural areas spent 2.8 times as much time on unpaid work as men, and those in urban areas spent 2.3 times more (National Bureau of Statistics of China 2019).

One area where gender equality outcomes have progressed is maternal healthcare. The maternal mortality rate has continued to decline, reaching 18.3 per 100,000 in 2018, which is commensurate with high-income countries. The urban-rural gap in maternal mortality was halved between 1990 and 2018. The rate of hospital delivery nationwide has increased substantially, reaching over 99% in both urban and rural areas. Institutional arrangements for "women's health protection" have brought better long-term health outcome and well-being to women (National Bureau of Statistics of China 2019). Girls' life expectancy at birth in 2020 was 79 years, an increase of 11 years from 1980; for boys in 2020, it was 75 years, an increase of 10 years from 1980 (World Bank 2019).

To provide enhanced legal protection of the physical and mental health of women and children, the Women's Rights and Protection Law, the Labor Law, the Marriage Law, the Minor Protection Law, the Anti-Domestic-Violence Law, the Special Provisions on Labor Protection for Female Employees, and the criminal law amendment to abolish prostitution of underage girls were all amended in 2020. These amendments are designed to include the development of government work plans to deliver on the health of key groups such as women, the elderly, and the disabled (Jiang 2020). What is observable here is that workplace and health laws are primary channels through which gender equality is being promoted. Most reform is devoted to ensuring that women can work but still carry out care duties at home, safely deliver children, and claim protection from violence as a "vulnerable" group.

In the emergency prevention, response, and recovery sector, decision-making power and authority rest with men. In China, a survey of men's and women's attitudes on vulnerability to climate change and disaster risks found that women have "less decision-making power on issues other than daily expenses" and "fewer opportunities to participate in their communities' public affairs" (Asia-Pacific Gender in Humanitarian Action Working Group 2020). Moreover, the representation of women in national and subnational discussions of disaster risk and reduction tends to position women as "vulnerable" rather than "active agents" (UN Women 2016).

In response to the COVID-19 pandemic, relevant government departments sought active participation from community-level civil society organizations, which are often women-focused and women-led. The government also provided support and care for frontline women healthcare staff and community workers (i.e., social workers, logisticians, civil society volunteers), prioritized pregnant women for medical treatment, and instituted protocols on the safety of pregnant women, mothers, and infants.

Personal hygiene packages were created for female medical staff, such as donated sanitary pad packages. These were promoted as reflecting the progress of Chinese society's understanding of gender and disaster emergency management (Zhou 2020). However, the "Mother's Mail Package" sent to pregnant women and the sanitary pad packages reveal a particular gendered narrative around who needs care and who delivers care. Mothers, for example, are a vulnerable group that should be assisted in providing care to others at home. Women healthcare workers may have periods, and this requires care, but their needs as workers, as decision-makers, and as mothers or wives were less promoted and were responded to with less organized care, as we will hear below.

Results

During the onset of the COVID-19 epidemic, most programs unrelated to COVID-19 were suspended. All staff in the public health sector and community sector (social welfare) were required to take on double shifts to continue working on routine tasks as well as assisting with the COVID-19 response. For CDC staff, some were relocated from Beijing to Wuhan, for example, for substantial periods of time. Almost all interviewees reported major changes in the nature of their tasks, working longer hours and being required to learn new skills to adapt to sudden changes. Most of those we interviewed expressed concern about the populations whose needs and safety may have been neglected or missed during the emergency.

Who Was Assigned to Crisis Response?

Women healthcare workers describe being required to do double shifts (this meant long hours), to agree to relocation (staying in hospitals or hotels), and experiencing periods of isolation when not on shift duty. All the women interviewed described how they were rarely in charge of the response in terms of decision-making. They followed orders rather than giving them.

> Our hospital is a public hospital, all the COVID-19 patients in the city were admitted to our hospital during the pandemic. We can't turn down COVID-19 patients. According to the requirements of the government, all patients must be admitted to our hospital. This is our responsibility as a designated hospital for infectious

diseases. Firstly, we must deal with all the administrative documents, including what our superior government departments require our hospital to do, and how we should guide [our] healthcare workers. (HCW3)

The proportion of women in the contaminated areas was relatively high, very high. Most of the wards in ICU were female nurses. Many doctors [mostly male] would stay in the doctor's office, which was a relatively clean area. In fact, doctors are more concerned with their cases, how to write medical records and discuss case files. For observing patients, nurses must have done the most. (HCW3)

For the staff in our department, when the epidemic came, we had to take tasks beyond our own workload. We obey the arrangement of the work unit. At the same time, we cannot ignore our own work. The superiors know about this, but we don't have other choices, we have to take care of both things, we have all been working very hard. (HCW1)

They also describe the double burden where, despite their physical removal from home, their care responsibilities remained. This sometimes created tension for women who wanted to be deployed but were unable to, due to family expectations to stay home and provide care. Others were not able to go home but were simultaneously expected by partners and family members to *be* home.

Especially true in [social] institutions like ours, female, mothers particularly, bears greater burden, for they need to take care of their kids. (CDC1)

But during the same times . . . I have to balance my family times and like for my work. So then I got some fire with my family like because it's like some kind of conflict, that's you cannot get out, if you go out there you cannot come back, so it's very disturbing at that time. (CSW4)

Women are always responsible for buying these things. I am the one in my family preparing things, masks, gloves, stuff like that. (HCW1)

Who Was Best Placed to Respond to Crisis?

Women and men assigned to surveillance, countermeasure, and coordination roles experienced a division of labor that was gendered rather than based on expertise, according to our women respondents. Highly knowledgeable and experienced women, especially in the CDC, were told that they could not be deployed on-site to conduct fieldwork investigations due to family carer roles and "personal needs."

Because I am female, and the male, that person, and . . . so they think they need to protect me. They think they have the responsibility to do the field investigation. I can stay in the office just to collect the data and analyze the data. It is easy for me. (CDC3)

> The pandemic has increased the burden on many women at home, as well as their role in the society. For example, the role as [frontline] healthcare workers, there are women who are working on environmental protection issues, and as community workers [i.e., social workers or civil society volunteers]. (CSW4)

> Actually, most of our leaders are men. So, in fact, a woman does not have a natural advantage . . . she will need to use more methods, good or bad. . . . In fact, it is women who stick it out and hang on out there in the end. (HCW3)

In some instances, these women were more senior in the organization than the men who were deployed. The women describe this as being strategic decision-making by those within the organization and explained that it would have consequences for their career progression compared to men. Some of the women described competition for clinical research resources because clinicians wanted to carve out a niche in the field during the pandemic by publishing the clinical research conducted on patients with COVID-19. Men colleagues frequently got ahead, with better chances to access the data and conduct research in clinical settings. When men were questioned about this, they would provide reasons such as the following:

> We have 24 rooms but they have one shower area, so you still can do that, just it will be a little bit . . . difficult for females. Like I will use five minutes to take a shower but for female normally they will use half an hour. This is not discrimination. Just the . . . we some time we think male, just that they are not so efficient. (HCW2)

> Although we have a lot of offices, so even female that also can live in office but mainly we will try to arrange male staff to work the outside because it will be a little convenient. (HCW2)

> Maybe, some women also have to work there [COVID-designated hospitals], but mostly we will try to arrange men staff to station in the hospitals. We also spent overnight in the hospital to work there. In this situation, we tried to arrange men to station at the hospital. We also stationed at the airport, most of the time, we arranged man to work in both places. (HCW1)

Impact on First Responders

Overwhelmingly, the women across all three sectors described how the emergency seemed to increase gender stereotyping. Each woman interviewee, regardless of sector, referred to the popular images of heroic masculinity compared to women as stressed, anxious, or in need.

> It [the pandemic] reinforces the traditional gender division of labor and gender phenomena. On the healthcare side, as people are increasingly seeing the [female]

> healthcare workers fighting against the pandemic, so maybe to a certain extent, it may have contributed to gender image reversal. But in general, it's just increased the burden and reinforced the roles of different sexes. (CSW2)

> During this epidemic we [women volunteers] not only help children with disability [in the community], but also other families, because they are faced with challenges, too. (CDC1)

What was unexpected is that some of the men we interviewed reported they felt stressed and anxious and were worried about their families but felt unable to express these feelings compared to women first responders.

> We are so tired. We usually work 10 to 12 hours a day. And mental stress is a problem for us. Our workplace support the mental care to the first line workers, including the healthcare workers, the epidemiologist workers and so forth. (CDC2)

> I'm in close contact with many cases at that time, so I'm worried if I go back to my home, maybe my children and my family members will catch the virus because of me. So I just stay outside. (HCW2)

> [Healthcare workers'] exposure and their risk of infection is indeed very high, as well as for family members of healthcare workers. Children [of healthcare workers] faced additional challenges and psychological distress because they are very worried about their parent(s) [working] at the front line. This also is a very difficult and very challenging stage, I think we are not doing enough, and they are in need of extra attention. (CSW1)

The few women who were not at home during the emergency describe having to manage perceptions that they were not good mothers because they were not at home to take on care roles.

> There is no good solution, the children can be sent to their grandparents or the dad or someone else who can help take care of them. After we explained the nature of our work to the teachers, they understood us better, and would often call my child. Teachers don't blame me too much for my child's poor homework or other reasons. (HCW1)

Other Observations

Finally, when we asked our participants to provide other observations that they felt were relevant to our research, some mentioned that they felt the social impact of the health emergency was not prioritized due to a lack of gender diversity among those in charge of emergency planning and response. Specific concerns raised were the escalation of violence at home and the permanent loss of income for women carers (i.e., for family members with disabilities). The responders who raised these concerns noted the absence of messaging and programs that recognized how some populations would be more vulnerable due to the public health interventions (i.e., lockdown).

> Before we did research that examined the increase of [violence] cases reported to local civil society organizations. But another official report didn't show the same. Our information doesn't match. But when you're worried about COVID-19, you don't have the time to report domestic violence because it's not the priority. (CSW2)

> During the pandemic, the cases of abuse coming to the one-stop center increased, and as you can imagine, in fact, most of the victims of sexual abuse are girls, we can see that more children were abused during the pandemic, the proportion of violence increased, because they are at home, they don't have any other places to go. (CSW1)

> If there is a child with disability in the family, the mother would basically not be able to work anymore for she doesn't have the time. Even if she had a job before and she had the ability to work, but she simply could not go to work. (CSW1)

Their concern was validated in our own interview experience. Contrast the concern about rising domestic violence incidents (first quote below) with the views of two senior officials interviewed for this project (second and third quotes below).

> I think during the lockdown period and the family members staying at home and they are all experiencing stress and uncertainty. So I think it's well, it's likely it's very likely to have more family violence against women, especially. (CSW2)

> Because lockdown means [that] the people are required to stay at home and they maybe more worried about the situation. Not violence. They don't have time to think about violençe. (HCW1)

> Frankly speaking, this situation [family violence] doesn't happen a lot in my province, so we don't put this in our meeting agenda. And this is not our primary source of problem, and what we want to prioritize is case detection, early detection and early response. (CSW3)

Findings and Conclusion

We noted above that existing research on first responders to the COVID-19 health emergency presents a (mostly) positive experience. We would not want our research to be interpreted as seeking to challenge or refute these accounts. Indeed, one respondent said that they felt more hopeful about the workplace culture after COVID-19, especially the workplace recognition of the need to balance work and care responsibilities.

In recent years, the Chinese government has progressed a range of gender equality laws to prohibit gender discrimination in the workplace, but social and political obstacles to gender inclusion remain high. In our interviews with those who were first responders in the first months of the COVID-19 outbreak in China, we find patterns of gendered division of labor among our interviewees. Nearly all women first responders we interviewed experienced the assignment of different tasks due to presumptions about women's endurance and mobility. Roles for first responders were assigned according to gender stereotypes, with women viewed as more susceptible to vulnerability and mental distress than men. Our interviews reveal enduring patterns of feminization and hegemonic masculinity that underpinned the crisis response. This was reflected not just in who was assigned to what tasks but also in the prioritization of secondary impacts that the crisis was having on communities. For example, senior leadership across the healthcare and community welfare sectors denied that domestic violence would be a concern during the pandemic despite evidence at the time of the interviews that this violence had risen dramatically. Gendered social norms determined who could best provide protection to others (women were seen as more fragile and dependent, whereas men were seen as stronger and independent [of family care duties]) and who could best provide care (women were seen as nurturers and caregivers, while men received care and made decisions). The experiences we describe in this chapter reveal the subtle, and not-so-subtle, gender dynamics of labor that were amplified during the COVID-19 crisis. As our respondents identified, it also amplified different experiences of recovery and assistance for populations affected by COVID-19 and emotional stress within the first responder population.

We note that as our sample was small, limited to those who were speaking in a professional capacity and concerned about being identified, we have not been able to draw meaningful conclusions about intersectional effects on frontline healthcare workers. This is a limitation that we are cognizant of, particularly when aware of our own position outside China at the time of writing. While we do not include demographic data for those we interviewed, we have attempted to integrate the underlying principals of intersectionality through questions focused on the structural barriers to equity and equality within institutions.

Our interviewees, without exception, referred to personal stress, anxiety, and sacrifice. These experiences, too, were gendered, with women first responders being expected to take orders, not give them, and to manage care obligations at work and home with little complaint. Men first responders, meanwhile, were expected to give orders, make decisions, and model mental strength to colleagues when it came to facing the risk of infection and separation from family. Women first responders, especially those associated with surveillance and clinical roles, were aware that being closer to the crisis was better for individuals' careers. They acknowledged in interviews that their male colleagues would benefit from being on the ground compared to the women, who had to stay in the office to process the data.

All interviewees referred to the stress of exposure to the virus, the change to working routines, and additional workloads. However, the three men interviewed noted that it was less acceptable for men to talk about stress, anxiety, or discomfort. The expectation was that they could be away from home and they would be less worried about infection.

All interviewees agreed that women first responders had to manage the double care burden more than men. The options for these women were minimal: manage work and home expectations without complaint but expect judgement (from partners, parents, and teachers); or stay home or at work (but not both). Those who went to work said that as the crisis went on, the judgement declined but they were aware of initial perceptions of them as neglectful mothers who put their children at risk of infection or did not come home each night. Finally, nine of our eleven interviewees raised their concern that vulnerable populations were neglected due to data and knowledge hierarchies. They described a situation where there was little interest or consideration of how the general population would manage additional health, economic and security risks during such a prolonged period of lockdown.

Our research suggests the need to prioritize gender inclusivity in health emergency preparation. This should include steps to mitigate the impact of infection measures and to engage in field experiment simulations that consider the management effects of equitable leadership representation and inclusion of gendered experiences during emergency response processes. There is a need for all public health and emergency response authorities to recognize the contribution of a sustained commitment to equity across the sectors responsible for disaster response and planning, and we recognize our own limitations in this regard. Finally, perceptions of what is "the priority" during the lockdown for families and individuals are informed by personal experiences, personal status, and gender identity among the first responders. In this case, first responders, for the most part, represent a highly educated, cis-gender, elite mainstream of urban Chinese society. China is not alone in having a first responder workforce that may not be representative of the groups who are most disproportionately disadvantaged during a crisis (Farhall et al. 2022). As such, though the findings we present here are unique to China and draw on the experiences of a select sample, they point to questions embedded in transnational feminist approaches around decision-making power, not only among genders but also across social locations, as well as the role of social norms and political context in structuring vulnerabilities.

References

Asia-Pacific Gender in Humanitarian Action Working Group. 2020. "The Covid-19 Outbreak and Gender: Key Advocacy Points from Asia and the Pacific." https://asiapacific.unwomen.org/sites/default/files/Field%20Office%20ESEAsia/Docs/Publications/2020/03/ap-GiHA-WG-advocacy.pdf.

Attané, Isabelle. 2012. "Being a Woman in China Today: A Demography of Gender," translated by Elizabeth Guill. *China Perspectives* (4): 5–15. https://doi.org/10.4000/chinaperspectives.6013.

Bishu, Sebawit, Sean McCandless, and Nicole Elias. 2021. "Gender in Emergency Services: Foundations for Greater Equity in Professional Codes of Ethics." *Public Integrity* 23 (6): 610–623. https://doi.org/10.1080/10999922.2020.1825179.

Braun, Virginia, and Victoria Clarke. 2013. *Successful Qualitative Research: A Practical Guide for Beginners*. London: SAGE.

Cao, Jinya, Jing Wei, Huadong Zhu, Yanping Duan, Wenqi Geng, Xia Hong, Jing Jiang, Xiaohui Zhao, and Boheng Zhu. 2020. "A Study of Basic Needs and Psychological Wellbeing of Medical Workers in the Fever Clinic of a Tertiary General Hospital in Beijing during the COVID-19 Outbreak." *Psychotherapy and Psychosomatics* 89 (4): 1–3. https://doi.org/10.1159/000507453.

Chappell, Louise, and Georgina Waylen. 2013. "Gender and the Hidden Life of Institutions." *Public Administration* 91 (3): 599–615. https://doi.org/10.1111/j.1467-9299.2012.02104.x.

Enarson, Elaine. 2012. *Women Confronting Natural Disaster: From Vulnerability to Resilience*. Boulder, CO: Lynne Rienner Publishers.

Farhall, Kate, Emma Gibson, and Niki Vincent. 2022. "Embedding Gender Equality in Emergency Management Planning." *Australian Journal of Emergency Management* 37 (1): 2.

Feng, Huiyun, Connie Cai Ru Gan, Diego Leiva, Bao Ling Zhang, and Sara E. Davies. 2022. "COVID-19, Sex, and Gender in China: A Scoping Review." *Globalization and Health* 18 (1): 1–12. https://doi.org/10.1186/s12992-022-00804-w.

Gan, Connie Cai Ru, Shuo Feng, Huiyun Feng, King-wa Fu, Sara E. Davies, Karen A. Grépin, Rosemary Morgan, Julia Smith, and Clare Wenham. 2022. "#WuhanDiary and #WuhanLockdown: Gendered Posting Patterns and Behaviours on Weibo during the COVID-19 Pandemic." *BMJ Global Health* 7 (4): e008149. https://doi.org/10.1136/bmjgh-2021-008149.

Gao, Hong, Adam Tyson, and Guangxin Cheng. 2022. "Novel Virus, Novel Response: Local Discretion and Responses to COVID-19 in Hebei Province, China." *Asia & the Pacific Policy Studies* 9 (1): 5–22. https://doi.org/10.1002/app5.342.

Gao, Xiaoyue, Lili Jiang, Yinqing Hu, Li Li, and Lili Hou. 2020. "Nurses' Experiences Regarding Shift Patterns in Isolation Wards during the COVID-19 Pandemic in China: A Qualitative Study." *Journal of Clinical Nursing* 29 (21–22): 4270–4280. https://doi.org/10.1111/jocn.15464.

International Labour Organization. 2017. "Improving Employment and Working Conditions in Health Services." International Labour Office. https://www.ilo.org/wcmsp5/groups/public/---ed_dialogue/---sector/documents/publication/wcms_548288.pdf.

Jiang, Xinhua. 2020. "Jinian "Beijing+25" Jiang Funv Jiankang Naru Juece Zhuliu Zhidu Baozhang Tixi Gengjia Chengshu Dingxing" [Commemorate Beijing+25: Mainstreaming Women's Health Decision-Making]. Xingbie Yanjiu Shiye [Gender Study and Perspective]. https://www.thepaper.cn/newsDetail_forward_8940972.

Liu, Yu-E., Zhong-Chang Zhai, Yan-Hong Han, Yi-Lan Liu, Feng-Ping Liu, and De-Ying Hu. 2020. "Experiences of Front-Line Nurses Combating Coronavirus Disease-2019 in China: A Qualitative Analysis." *Public Health Nursing* 37 (5): 757–763. https://doi.org/10.1111/phn.12768.

Long, Yan. 2018. "The Contradictory Impact of Transnational AIDS Institutions on State Repression in China, 1989–2013." *American Journal of Sociology* 124 (2): 309–366. https://doi.org/10.1086/698466.

National Bureau of Statistics of China. 2019. "Women and Men in China: Facts and Figures 2019." Department of Social, Science, Technology and Cultural Statistics, National Bureau of Statistics. https://cnlgbtdata.com/files/uploads/2020/01/%E4%B8%AD%E5%9B%BD%E7%A4%BE%E4%BC%9A%E4%B8%AD%E7%9A%84%E5%A5%B3%E4%BA%BA%E5%92%8C%E7%94%B7%E4%BA%BA2019EN-final.pdf.

Qing, Shisong. 2020. "Gender Role Attitudes and Male-Female Income Differences in China." *Journal of Chinese Sociology* 7 (1): 12. https://doi.org/10.1186/s40711-020-00123-w.

Ren, Annie. 2022. "How the "Garlic Chives" Grieved: A Song for China's Three-Child Policy." In *China Story Yearbook: Contradiction*, edited by Esther Sunkyung Klein, Linda Jaivin, and Sharon Strange, 171–177. Canberra, Australia: ANU Press. https://doi.org/10.22459/CSY.2022.05A.

Smith, Julia, Sara E. Davies, Huiyun Feng, Connie C. R. Gan, Karen A. Grépin, Sophie Harman, Asha Herten-Crabb, Rosemary Morgan, Nimisha Vandan, and Clare Wenham. 2021. "More than a Public Health Crisis: A Feminist Political Economic Analysis of COVID-19." *Global Public Health* 16 (8–9): 1–17. https://doi.org/10.1080/17441692.2021.1896765.

Song, Lin. 2021. "Straightly Chinese: The Emergence of Systemic Homophobia in China." In *Contesting Chineseness: Ethnicity, Identity, and Nation in China and Southeast Asia*, edited by Chang-Yau Hoon and Ying-kit Chan, 305–317. Singapore: Springer Nature. https://doi.org/10.1007/978-981-33-6096-9_16.

Sun, Wenxiu, Wei-Ti Chen, Qing Zhang, Siyue Ma, Feifei Huang, Lin Zhang, and Hongzhou Lu. 2021. "Post-Traumatic Growth Experiences among COVID-19 Confirmed Cases in China: A Qualitative Study." *Clinical Nursing Research* 30 (7): 1079–1087. https://doi.org/10.1177/10547738211016951.

UN Women. 2016. "Gender Dimensions of Vulnerability to Climate Change in China." https://asiapacific.unwomen.org/en/digital-library/publications/2016/12/gender-dimensions-of-vulnerability-to-climate-change-in-china.

Wenham, Clare, Julia Smith, and Rosemary Morgan. 2020. "COVID-19: The Gendered Impacts of the Outbreak." *Lancet* 395 (10227): 846–848. https://doi.org/10.1016/S0140-6736(20)30526-2.

WHO. 2022. "China: WHO Coronavirus Disease (COVID-19) Dashboard with Vaccination Data." *World Health Organization*. https://data.who.int/dashboards/covid19/cases.

World Bank. 2019. "Survival to Age 65, Female (% of Cohort)—China." United Nations Population Division, World Population Prospects. https://data.worldbank.org/indicator/SP.DYN.TO65.FE.ZS?locations=CN.Zhou, Yuan. 2020. "Jinian 'Beijing+25' Xin Xingshi Xia de Zhongguo Huanjing Baohu yu Funv" [Commemorate Beijing +25: China's Environmental Protection and Women under the New Normal]. Xingbie Yanjiu Shiye [Gender Study and Perspective]. https://m.thepaper.cn/newsDetail_forward_9079453.

6 "We Want to Improve the Situation, but It's Not under Our Control": Gendered Risks, Impacts, and Response in Hong Kong

Ingrid D. Lui and Karen A. Grépin

Introduction

The Hong Kong Special Administrative Region (hereafter Hong Kong) is an East Asian society that was home to 7.5 million people as of the end of 2019. COVID-19 policies took effect in Hong Kong in early January 2020, when the government first began to respond to the reports of a cluster of viral pneumonias of unknown etiology in Wuhan, China. By the end of 2022, Hong Kong had experienced five distinct waves of COVID-19 outbreaks, with the first two of those waves being relatively mild and taking place between January and April 2020. The third wave of infections took place between July and September 2020, and the fourth wave began in late November 2020 and concluded around April 2021. Hong Kong enjoyed a long period of zero locally transmitted cases until the fifth wave began in early 2022, triggered by the Omicron variant. By December 31, 2022, Hong Kong had reported a cumulative total of 2.60 million COVID-19 cases and 11,807 deaths (Worldometer 2024).

Hong Kong's approach to the COVID-19 pandemic was relatively unique, as it was one of the few places in the world to continue pursuing a "dynamic zero-COVID" strategy through 2022. Through strict measures such as contact tracing, border controls, and mass testing exercises, the goal of this strategy was to prevent new outbreaks from occurring by quickly identifying cases as they arose, ultimately keeping the number of local infections to zero. Mindful of the recent history of severe acute respiratory syndrome (SARS), travel restrictions were quickly imposed in January 2020 to restrict travelers from mainland China, and these were soon extended to all inbound travelers who were not Hong Kong residents. Throughout the pandemic, passenger flights from high-risk locations specified by the government were regularly banned, and all travelers needed to undergo a minimum fourteen-day quarantine period upon their arrival at home, in a hotel or at a government quarantine center.

Similarly, the government passed an array of policies to prevent the transmission of COVID-19 in the community. Under the Prevention and Control of Disease Ordinance, which existed prior to the COVID-19 pandemic, members of the public were required to wear masks in public spaces and limits were imposed on the number of people who could gather in public spaces. Limits were also imposed on the number of people who could occupy tables at dine-in restaurants. Furthermore, school closures were instituted on and off throughout the pandemic, particularly during the peaks of infection waves, with students learning either fully online or in person on a half-day basis. Overall, and especially early in the pandemic, many praised Hong Kong's response to COVID as being incredibly effective to maintain low case numbers and limit deaths (Gibney 2020). However, it seems that feminist perspectives were not taken into consideration during the planning and implementation of these policies, given the socioeconomic impacts on women we will discuss in more detail later in this chapter.

Prior to the COVID-19 pandemic, the Hong Kong government implemented several initiatives to promote gender equality. The Equal Opportunities Commission, established in 1996, serves to eliminate discrimination and harassment of, and promote equal opportunities for, individuals irrespective of sex, disability, family status, and race. It is also responsible for upholding the Sexual Discrimination Ordinance, which states that it is unlawful to discriminate against someone because of their sex in areas such as employment and education. The Women's Commission was established in 2001 to oversee women's concerns, develop long-term strategies that promote women's empowerment, and advise the government on policies and initiatives that concern women. The Gender Mainstreaming Checklist was developed to encourage government officers to take different gender-related needs and views into consideration during the policymaking process. In practice, however, Hong Kong still has a long way to go before achieving gender equality both in policy and beyond. A coalition of local women's groups previously conducted a study of the implementation of gender mainstreaming in Hong Kong, concluding that the Women's Commission did not have the authority to influence government policies and that the Gender Mainstreaming Checklist's effectiveness was questionable given the inadequacy of gender-related training and unsystematic usage of the checklist (Chan and Kan 2017). Even in the post-COVID world, one of the coalition members, the Hong Kong Federation of Women's Centres, continues to call for the government to promote gender mainstreaming to improve local women's mental health and quality of life (University of Hong Kong 2024), suggesting that little has changed from a policy perspective since their previous study.

Hong Kong has several cultural barriers that enforce specific gender roles for men and women. The patriarchal nature of Hong Kong society means that childcare is still viewed as primarily women's work that is carried out exclusively by the family rather than shared by the state (Leung 2018). As such, the lack of social support for childcare and gendered perceptions of caring duties creates a double burden for working mothers, especially low-income mothers who are unable to afford childcare services (Leung 2018). Gender stereotypes, including traditional gender role expectations, are seen by both members of the public and political leaders as a barrier for women to attain leadership positions (Song et al. 2020). Additionally, there is a view that gender discrimination is not an issue in Hong Kong, which may be partially based on women's increased participation in occupations traditionally held by men, such as medicine and politics (Schnurr and Mak 2011). In Hong Kong, the lack of gender-sensitive initiatives at a policy level, as well as patriarchal social norms, created an environment where gender issues were not readily discussed even before the pandemic.

Through the Gender & COVID-19 project, a Hong Kong research team sought to understand how economic, health and educational policy responses to COVID-19 in Hong Kong affected men and women differently, particularly those women positioned at the intersection of multiple structural inequities. When COVID-19 first emerged, researchers and policymakers in the city were primarily focused on understanding the novel virus and preventing its transmission, with little consideration of the downstream socioeconomic effects on the public, let alone the unique effects the pandemic would have on women and other disadvantaged communities. Toward the end of the pandemic, in late 2022, research emerged that discussed some of the socioeconomic consequences of pandemic-era measures, including a discussion of "COVID social risks" by Choi et al. (2022) and the health impacts and life challenges faced by Hong Kong Chinese women by Hung et al. (2022). However, the former only discussed issues such as employment and income or care at a broader level for comparison with the situations in South Korea and

Taiwan (Choi, Kühner, and Shi 2022), while the latter only focused on Hong Kong Chinese women and therefore did not include any analyses of ethnic minority women's experiences (Hung, Chan, and Liu 2022). Therefore, our research aims to further contribute to this literature on the lived experiences of women in Hong Kong during COVID-19.

In this chapter, we explore economic, health, educational, and quarantine and testing policy responses from the perspectives of those women most affected, namely those located at the intersections of multiple inequities, including those in precarious work or with low incomes, healthcare workers, mothers, and women from ethnic minorities. By taking this transnational feminist lived-experience approach to policy analysis, we aim to illuminate how global and local structural inequities disadvantaged and overburdened these women in Hong Kong throughout the COVID-19 response, imposing disproportionate negative effects.

Methods

We conducted interviews with affected constituencies as identified by the COVID-19 and Gender Matrix (Morgan et al. 2022; Smith et al. 2021), including healthcare professionals, low-income and precariously employed women, mothers, and ethnic minority women to illustrate how different demographic groups with intersecting drivers of inequality were affected by the COVID-19 pandemic, particularly in relation to gender. Between May and October 2020, we conducted interviews with fifty-two women and eighteen men affected by the pandemic over the phone or via Zoom. Respondents worked in a variety of occupations, including foreign domestic workers,[1] healthcare professionals, and nongovernmental organization (NGO) staff. Most of the interviews were carried out by one researcher and were conducted in English. Five interviews were conducted in Urdu, and one in Hindi by that same researcher, who is fluent in both languages. One interview was conducted in Cantonese by a different researcher, who is a native speaker. All foreign-language interviews were subsequently translated into English by the respective interviewer. All interviews were analyzed using framework analysis, again based on the COVID-19 and Gender Matrix, to identify groups of women particularly affected by specific policies and gain their perspectives on that aspect of the pandemic response.

The Health Policy Response as Experienced by Healthcare Workers

The robust public health response to COVID-19 in Hong Kong created unique demands on healthcare workers. In February 2020, the public hospital system reduced its provision of nonessential and nonemergency services to shift staff and resources toward combating the epidemic (Government of the Hong Kong Special Administrative Region 2020a). The government converted AsiaWorld-Expo, Hong Kong's largest exhibition and event venue, into a makeshift COVID-19 treatment facility in August 2020 (Ting 2020) and built new facilities such as a quarantine center in Penny's Bay (news.gov.hk 2020). Furthermore, they introduced several COVID-19 testing initiatives, such as the two-week voluntary Universal Community Testing Program in September 2020 (Government of the Hong Kong Special Administrative Region 2020b).

Our healthcare worker participants, including ten nurses and six doctors, noted that the pandemic led to numerous changes in how health services were prioritized and used by the public. Due to the reduction of nonessential services, appointments had to be rescheduled as patients either found it difficult to attend their follow-ups or chose not to go at all for fear of infection, which continued to cause chaos for the healthcare system. Additionally, patients tended to avoid going to the hospital when cases were high, with one woman doctor working in the public sector describing "a huge rush of people coming back to clinic to make up for the appointments that they had missed" once the number of cases subsided, causing difficulties for healthcare staff working in an already overwhelmed system. As another public sector woman doctor explained, "A lot of our patients require multidisciplinary care . . . and if they're not getting the care that they need, we can't coordinate."

Healthcare worker participants also recalled COVID-19 patients who would act aggressively toward them, such as yelling at them or refusing to follow their instructions. One of the main worries expressed by women healthcare workers caring for COVID-19 patients was that they might get exposed to the virus and how this would affect their family members, particularly those living with elderly parents or infants. This was a valid concern, particularly during the initial months of the pandemic when frontline healthcare workers reported inadequate access to personal protective equipment (Chau et al. 2021). In addition to physical risk, fear of infection posed a major mental burden, especially as workers feared they could be asymptomatic carriers of COVID-19. One woman nurse explained that she was hesitant to go for voluntary COVID-19 testing because "I'm afraid I already got infected . . . and we don't know what [consequences that] would bring."

Hong Kong's public hospitals were already experiencing a staffing shortage problem prior to the pandemic, but this became more pronounced as staff were reallocated to serve on the front lines. At the same time, human resource shortages were further compounded by women leaving the workforce to spend more time caring for their families (we will also elaborate on the impact on women from other professions in the section on education below). As one male doctor observed,

> During the early COVID outbreak, I know that some of the female staff in the public [hospital] system quit their job. I think because they think themselves is the family carer and they foresee it will affect their children or affect their families so they will take up the family caring role.

Overall, women healthcare workers were not consulted about the changes to the health system, though they had to deal with the consequences. This is perhaps best captured by the following two quotes:

> It would be more valuable if there is some authority [who] can reach out actively and then ask what do we need and what do we want or what kind of assistance we need. . . . I think there should be some more interaction in two ways but not only one way. (woman, NGO nurse)

> The burden of controlling a pandemic should not fall on the frontline staff or the general populace, it should fall at a government level and a policy level, and certainly they haven't been doing that. (woman, public sector doctor)

Economic Policy Response as Experienced by Lower-Income and Precariously Employed Women

The pandemic had many effects on women's work and financial situations, particularly as the sectors that were heavily affected by pandemic-related job losses, such as hospitality, primarily employ women, and women make up the majority of low-income and precariously employed workers in Hong Kong (Oxfam 2017). For example, a woman private tutor who worked on contract, and whose husband recently lost his job while she lost a large portion of her clients, said,

> I think we really cannot do too much to improve the situation, because a lot of the employers are not recruiting workers. . . . So this is quite difficult for us, it's like we want to improve the situation, but it's not our choice, it's not under our control.

Participants reported job losses, reduced working hours, and being forced to take leave without pay. Those who worked in essential services such as cleaning work, who are often ethnic minorities living in poverty, were unable to work from home and thus may have been at a higher risk of income loss. For example, one male, ethnic minority street cleaner described how "more people are coming for work but there is less money . . . so many people work for two shifts." He also described a cycle of work and illness, where "all workers here are sick. They have pain but they do not have time to go to hospital."

Recognizing the economic effects of its strict physical distancing policies, the Hong Kong government offered some financial assistance to each eligible Hong Kong permanent resident age eighteen or above, with an HKD (Hong Kong dollars) 10,000 (USD 1,275) cash disbursement in July 2020 and consumption vouchers issued via e-payment platforms in August 2021. It also provided subsidies to companies affected by the pandemic response so they could retain their workforce. While respondents were grateful for such support, those who lost their jobs or had their work temporarily suspended were worried about their future job situation and struggled to find new employment. Some complained that the government's payments were often limited or only one-off, and they questioned how long the payments would last, particularly for low-income individuals and households. Participants whose companies received financial assistance also felt that the money benefitted the company more than the employees. Those who relied on government assistance, such as the Comprehensive Social Security Assistance Scheme, stressed that it alone was not enough to cover their day-to-day expenses. Similar criticisms were expressed of the HKD 10,000 cash payout scheme, with some participants questioning how far it could reasonably support low-income individuals. The lack of income made it even more difficult to afford necessities such as food and rent, a burden that was compounded by increasing prices around the city. A woman special needs educator explained, "The government didn't give you anything other than the 10,000 dollar[s] for everyone. Other than that, you have just to survive on your own."

Low-income ethnic minority families were more likely to face job losses and salary cuts (Diocesan Pastoral Centre for Workers—Ethnic Minorities Service 2020), making it more difficult for them to pay for necessities. They also faced difficulties in applying for financial aid and needed to seek help from community organizations to do so. Foreign workers, including foreign domestic workers, were specifically excluded from government financial support, even though they faced increased pressure to send money back home to their families and would have benefited greatly from the assistance.

Educational Policy Response as Experienced by Mothers

Hong Kong instituted some of the longest and most frequent COVID-19-related school closures—over ten months in total during the first two years of the pandemic. Due to the gender norms described above, the burden of caring for children attending school virtually at home fell particularly on mothers, with notable effects on their careers and well-being. The mothers we interviewed who had to work from home during the pandemic found it difficult to do so with young children around. Many described how women were facing increased care responsibilities at home, including making sure their children were focused during online lessons or taking care of husbands who stayed home to work. A mom and NGO worker observed,

> I would say that women have also had to deal with the brunt of having children at home and being in charge of them and their education and trying to figure things out. . . . Their mental state has been so poorly impacted by COVID.

Mothers worried greatly about the well-being of their children due to a lack of opportunities to socialize with others. Some noted that educational progress was stalled due to difficulties transitioning to online learning and focusing during class as well as a lack of access to in-person support from their schools and teachers. Mothers feared that the lack of social interaction would cause their child's emotional development to suffer, with younger children acting more emotionally volatile (e.g., being quick to anger) and older children becoming more isolated. One ethnic minority single mother said, "I understand [the outbreak], I had been going through [it]. But the children don't understand. And it becomes a part of their personality and it can worsen their adult life."

In response, some mothers turned to networks of community support to share resources and information, including community organizations as well as friends and family. However, the overall stress of trying to both manage professional commitments and ensure their children's educational development and well-being weighed on mothers.

Compulsory Quarantine and Testing as Experienced by Ethnic Minority Women

Although our team had stopped conducting interviews by October 2020, there were several policies that came into effect afterward that warrant discussion. The Hong Kong government introduced compulsory testing notices in late November 2020, where people who were present in a specified location at the same time as a confirmed COVID-19 patient were required to undergo a COVID-19 test by a given deadline at a community testing center. The next iteration of this policy was the restriction-testing declarations introduced in December 2020, which prevented people from entering or leaving certain premises unless they could show a negative COVID-19 test result. This was often imposed on residential buildings, with government teams dispatched to specific locations to test all residents or having them visit a temporary testing tent. Specific testing policies also appeared to target ethnic minorities.

On April 30, 2021, the government declared that all foreign domestic workers in Hong Kong, a group of around 370,000 people primarily made up of women from Southeast Asian countries such as the Philippines, were required to undergo compulsory COVID-19 testing. This decision was in response to two foreign domestic workers who had recently tested positive. The government justified this decision by highlighting the nature of the workers' jobs as caregivers in family settings who could affect their employer's family members if they got infected (news.gov.hk 2021). Although this first round of testing ended on May 9, a second round of compulsory testing was announced on May 12, taking place from May 15 to May 30. If foreign domestic workers failed to comply, they would be fined a fixed penalty of HKD 5,000 (USD 638).

The foreign domestic workers interviewed during the third wave previously expressed that these policies were particularly blind to this group's unique experiences and needs despite targeting them directly (Lui et al. 2021), and it seems that this testing mandate was no exception. Although other occupational groups were also subject to mandatory testing arrangements based on the riskiness of their jobs (e.g., restaurant workers or teachers), the rationale provided for foreign domestic workers was based more on the perceived riskiness of activities and behaviors they engaged in during their rest days, such as large group gatherings with friends in public spaces (Lui and Grépin 2021b). Furthermore, the Hong Kong government repeatedly treated this group as needing oversight to control their actions in order to protect themselves and others against COVID-19, yet foreign domestic workers had demonstrated their willingness to seek out health information and get vaccinated even without the support from the government (Lui and Grépin 2021a).

On January 23, 2021, a new form of restriction was introduced along with targeted testing, known colloquially as "ambush lockdowns." Without warning, residents of a four-block radius in the Jordan district—a densely populated area that was home to a large ethnic minority community—were confined to their homes for forty-eight hours and had to undergo mandatory testing for COVID-19; the lockdown was only lifted once all residents had been tested. For the next two weeks, until the Chinese New Year holiday, this type of lockdown occurred nearly every day, with the official goal of identifying cases early and preventing transmission chains from occurring in buildings that were often old and overcrowded. However, this practice was largely divisive among the community; some questioned the cost-effectiveness of testing thousands of people only to yield very few, if any, positive results, whereas others felt this was necessary to ensure that an area had zero infections (Davidson 2021). After May 2022, the government continued to issue restriction and testing declarations on buildings with positive cases but stopped "ambushing" the targeted locations.

From a gender perspective, these ambush lockdowns created a huge amount of stress on the residents of the targeted buildings. Since the goal of these lockdowns was to not alert residents in advance so that they could not leave the building ahead of time, they created a lot of anxiety for Hong Kong people, wondering if their building would be next. As women are likely to be responsible for running the household (e.g., planning meals, even if a foreign domestic worker is the one to prepare them), this uncertainty created more pressure for them to ensure that their family would be prepared if a lockdown was enforced, especially as the government did not provide essentials such as food or hygiene supplies for locked-down residents. Furthermore, as these lockdowns prevented people from leaving home to go to work, those who could not work from home (as discussed above) likely suffered from the pay they missed during the lockdown. Finally, although these lockdowns were relatively short and lasted between twelve and forty-eight hours, it is still important to note that lockdown measures have the potential to increase rates of domestic violence and prevent women from accessing help (Wenham et al. 2020).

Discussion

From our participants' lived experiences of the pandemic up to October 2020, particularly during the third wave of infections, several patterns emerge about the gendered effects of COVID-19 in Hong Kong. The workload of both paid and unpaid care was felt to have greatly increased during the pandemic, a burden that was overwhelmingly placed on women. For example, as more children were forced to stay home during government-mandated school closures, women were generally expected to care for them, even if they had full-time work to attend to at the same time. As mentioned previously, childcare has historically not been seen as the government's responsibility, which may have prevented the government from working with schools to provide adequate support for students and their caregivers. This effect can also be seen in the impact on the healthcare system, where little assistance seemed to be provided to the frontline staff of the healthcare sector to ease their burden.

Additionally, the policies that were brought in during this time to mitigate the downstream effects of COVID-19 were mostly blind to their potential gendered effects and thus greatly disadvantaged women already marginalized. One key example of this is the one-off HKD 10,000 cash payout scheme, which failed to sufficiently support some of the city's most vulnerable women while also excluding other groups entirely, such as foreign domestic workers, who are primarily women. As such, for this group of women in Hong Kong, the inequalities and discrimination that existed for them long before the pandemic continued to affect how they were treated by the government and society at large. This speaks to broader trends of global capitalist systems of power and privilege creating transnational structures and policies that disadvantage the most vulnerable migrant women of color. As such, from this systemic perspective it shares much in common with chapters 3, 4, and 8. Not only did the government fail to prioritize the needs of those made most vulnerable, but it seems that policies were not considered from a gender-based perspective despite the existence of the Gender Mainstreaming

Checklist. These patterns, unfortunately, continued throughout the course of the pandemic, including during the fourth wave of infections, which occurred shortly after our interviews concluded.

Other policies indicate deeply embedded structural racism. For instance, ethnic minority women were particularly singled out by enforced quarantine and testing policies. Foreign domestic workers were required to get tested despite already high compliance with public health measures, and neighborhoods known to house ethnic minorities were subjected to ambush-style lockdowns. Evidence from previous lockdowns suggests women bore the cost of such lockdowns in terms of both their economic and physical security. That no efforts were made by the government to directly mitigate secondary effects of the policies introduced to limit COVID-19's spread on racialized women and other vulnerable groups within Hong Kong society reveals much in relation to the patriarchal dominance within the administration.

Although the focus of this research is primarily on the gendered effects of the COVID-19 pandemic, the Hong Kong case highlights the importance of taking an intersectional approach to policy analysis. As of the 2021 population census, 8.4 percent of the population, including foreign domestic workers, was of non-Chinese ethnicity, with 78.7 percent of them being non-Chinese Asians (Census and Statistics Department 2022). Despite this, half of our interviewees were ethnic minorities, as we felt that their experiences would not be heard if we had taken a more representative approach to sampling. In recent years, more studies have been emerging out of Hong Kong that use an intersectional approach to investigate issues affecting women, and migrant women more specifically. For example, Hung et al. (2020) reanalyzed evaluation data from a women's empowerment community project using an intersectional lens and discussed how low-income migrant women were more likely to question traditional gender norms based on the experiences they encountered at the intersection of their gender, race, and class. This study therefore contributes to this growing body of literature by demonstrating the unique experiences ethnic minority women faced during the COVID-19 pandemic.

Conclusion

The story of the COVID-19 pandemic in Hong Kong up until June 2021 has demonstrated the near-universal truth that women around the world are facing numerous structural inequalities that are being exposed by social policies introduced to mitigate the pandemic. This is particularly true for ethnic minority women (including foreign domestic workers) and working women with families, who have faced the brunt of caring responsibilities and strict testing policies. Furthermore, the Hong Kong government has done little to consider the gendered impacts of the policies they introduce, though this is sadly in line with the broader gendered discourse in Hong Kong that predates the pandemic. Thus, the Hong Kong case study demonstrates that, even in a context where gender inequality is not considered as an important policy area, the COVID-19 pandemic has exposed that gender equality is very much still an issue in Hong Kong public policy.

Note

1. For a more detailed analysis of the data on foreign domestic workers from this project, please see Lui et al. (2021).

References

Census and Statistics Department. 2022. "Thematic Report: Ethnic Minorities." Census and Statistics Department. https://www.censtatd.gov.hk/en/data/stat_report/product/B1120111/att/B11201112021XXXXB0100.pdf.

Chan, Hau Nung, and Man Ki Kan. 2017. "Research Report of Implementation of Gender Mainstreaming in Hong Kong" [in Chinese]. Hong Kong Women's Coalition on Equal Opportunities. https://womencentre.org.hk/En/Newsroom/publication/Upload/article/35/Download/5e21598e2da9f.pdf.

Chau, Janita Pak Chun, Suzanne Hoi Shan Lo, Ravneet Saran, Claudia Ho Yau Leung, Simon Kwun Yu Lam, and David R. Thompson. 2021. "Nurses' Experiences of Caring for People with COVID-19 in Hong Kong: A Qualitative Enquiry." *BMJ Open* 11 (8): e052683. https://doi.org/10.1136/bmjopen-2021-052683.

Choi, Young Jun, Stefan Kühner, and Shih-Jiunn Shi. 2022. "From 'New Social Risks' to 'COVID Social Risks': The Challenges for Inclusive Society in South Korea, Hong Kong, and Taiwan Amid the Pandemic." *Policy and Society* 41 (2): 260–274. https://doi.org/10.1093/polsoc/puac001.

Davidson, Helen. 2021. "'Ambush' Lockdowns: Hong Kong Tries Radical COVID Testing Strategy." *The Guardian*, February 3. https://www.theguardian.com/world/2021/feb/03/ambush-lockdowns-hong-kong-tries-radical-covid-testing-strategy.

Diocesan Pastoral Centre for Workers—Ethnic Minorities Service. 2020. "Report on the Employment Situation of Local Ethnic Minorities (EMs) during the Outbreak of COVID-19 Epidemic." Hong Kong: Catholic Diocese of Hong Kong. https://www.hkccla.org.hk/article/RI_20201120.pdf.

Gibney, Elizabeth. 2020. "Whose Coronavirus Strategy Worked Best? Scientists Hunt Most Effective Policies." *Nature* 581: 15–16. https://doi.org/10.1038/d41586-020-01248-1.

Government of the Hong Kong Special Administrative Region. 2020a. "HA Adjusts Service Provision to Focus on Combatting Epidemic." Press release, February 10. https://www.info.gov.hk/gia/general/202002/10/P2020021000711.htm.

Government of the Hong Kong Special Administrative Region. 2020b. "Summary of Results of the Universal Community Testing Programme." Press release, September 15. https://www.info.gov.hk/gia/general/202009/15/P2020091500931.htm.

Hung, Maria Shuk Yu, Liliane Chui King Chan, and Sisi Pui Shan Liu. 2022. "The Health Impacts and Life Challenges Caused by the COVID-19 Pandemic on Hong Kong Chinese Women." *International Journal of Environmental Research and Public Health* 19 (19): 5115. https://doi.org/10.3390/ijerph19095115.

Hung, Suet-lin, Kwok-kin Fung, and Siu-mei Lau. 2020. "Intersectionality and Gender: Community Practice with Low-Income Migrant Women." *Community Development Journal* 55 (1): 102–120. https://doi.org/10.1093/cdj/bsz026.

Leung, Lai-ching. 2018. "Gender Matters: Rethinking the Childcare Model in Hong Kong." *Children & Society* 32 (5): 393–404. https://doi.org/10.1111/chso.12260.

Lui, Ingrid, and Karen Grépin. 2021a. "Understanding COVID-19 Vaccination Rates among Hong Kong's Foreign Domestic Workers." *Gender & COVID-19* (blog), May 5. https://www.genderandcovid-19.org/editorial/understanding-covid-19-vaccination-rates-among-hong-kongs-foreign-domestic-workers/.

Lui, Ingrid, and Karen A. Grépin. 2021b. "Why Hong Kong's Policy Response to COVID-19 Doesn't Work for Foreign Domestic Workers." *Gender & COVID-19* (blog). November 13. https://www.genderandcovid-19.org/editorial/why-hong-kongs-policy-response-to-covid-19-doesnt-work-for-foreign-domestic-workers/.

Lui, Ingrid D., Nimisha Vandan, Sara E. Davies, Sophie Harman, Rosemary Morgan, Julia Smith, Clare Wenham, and Karen Ann Grépin. 2021. "'We Also Deserve Help During the Pandemic': The Effect of the COVID-19 Pandemic on Foreign Domestic Workers in Hong Kong." *Journal of Migration and Health* 3: 100037. https://doi.org/10.1016/j.jmh.2021.100037.

Morgan, Rosemary, Sara E. Davies, Huiyin Feng, Connie C. R. Gan, Karen A. Grépin, Sophie Harman, Asha Herten-Crabb, Julia Smith, and Clare Wenham. 2022. "Using Gender Analysis Matrixes to Integrate a Gender Lens into Infectious Diseases Outbreaks Research." *Health Policy and Planning* 37 (7) (August): 935–941. https://doi.org/10.1093/heapol/czab149.

news.gov.hk. 2020. "CS Inspects New Quarantine Units." Press release, July 13. https://www.news.gov.hk/eng/2020/07/20200713/20200713_180838_810.html.

news.gov.hk. 2021. "Helper Virus Testing Explained." Press release, May 1. https://www.news.gov.hk/eng/2021/05/20210501/20210501_221318_805.html.

Oxfam. 2017. "Executive Summary: Research on Low-Income Casual Work in Hong Kong." https://www.oxfam.org.hk/en/f/news_and_publication/1408/content_34010en.pdf.

Schnurr, Stephanie, and Bernie Mak. 2011. "Leadership in Hong Kong. Is Gender Really Not an Issue?" *Gender and Language* 5 (2): 343–371. https://doi.org/10.1558/genl.v5i2.343.

Smith, Julia, Sara E. Davies, Huiyin Feng, Connie C. R. Gan, Karen A. Grépin, Sophie Harman, Asha Herten-Crabb, et al. 2021. "More Than a Public Health Crisis: A Feminist Political Economic Analysis of COVID-19." *Global Public Health* 16 (8–9): 1364–1380. https://doi.org/10.1080/17441692.2021.1896765.

Song, Jing, Sally Ka-wing Lo, Haijing Dai, Anthony Ying-him Fung, Ching-man Lam, and Fanny M. Cheung. 2020. "A Study on Public Attitudes Towards Female Political Leadership." Gender Research Centre, Hong Kong Institute of Asia-Pacific Studies, The Chinese University of Hong Kong. https://www.eoc.org.hk/EOC/upload/ResearchReport/20201007ResearchReport_MainReport_E.pdf.

Ting, Victor. 2020. "Coronavirus: 400 beds Likely to Be Ready at Hong Kong's AsiaWorld-Expo by This Week, Hospital Authority Says." *South China Morning Post*, August 11. https://www.scmp.com/news/hong-kong/health-environment/article/3096965/coronavirus-400-beds-likely-be-ready-hong-kongs.

University of Hong Kong. 2024. "Survey Findings on 'Women's Quality of Life and Public's Attitude toward Gender Equality in Hong Kong.'" Press release, March 4. https://www.hku.hk/press/press-releases/detail/27115.html.

Wenham, Clare, Julia Smith, Sara E. Davies, Huiyin Feng, Karen A. Grépin, Sophie Harman, Asha Herten-Crabb, and Rosemary Morgan. 2020. "Women Are Most Affected by Pandemics—Lessons from Past Outbreaks." *Nature* 583: 194–198. https://doi.org/10.1038/d41586-020-02006-z.

Worldometer. 2024. "Hong Kong COVID—Coronavirus Statistics." Last modified March 26. https://www.worldometers.info/coronavirus/country/china-hong-kong-sar/.

7 "Since They Call Us Volunteers, There Is No Support at All": Community Health Volunteers during the COVID-19 Pandemic in Kenya

Anne Ngunjiri, Robinson Karuga, Linet Okoth, and Lillian Otiso

Introduction

In Kenya, the first case of COVID-19 was identified on March 13, 2020. Soon after the announcement of the virus in the country (on February 19, 2020), the Kenyan government, through the Ministry of Health (MoH), put several preventive measures in place to curb its transmission and adverse effects on the public. The multiagency National Emergency Response Committee on Coronavirus coordinated the implementation of these measures, and the MoH released protocols and guidelines outlining individual, household, and community interventions and preventive measures to be observed. These included COVID-19 screening and testing, isolation and quarantine, physical distancing restrictions, movement restrictions and lockdowns in counties with high COVID-19 burdens, curfews, and school closures (Aluga 2020; Barasa et al. 2021; Wangari et al. 2021).

The measures to contain COVID-19 had dire consequences on the lives and livelihoods of Kenyan households (World Bank Group 2021). These include job losses, business and school disruptions, and economic and poverty-related stress and food insecurity (Mueller, Grépin, et al. 2022; Mueller, Ngunjiri, et al. 2022; Oyando et al. 2021; Pinchoff et al. 2021). According to the Kenya National Bureau of Statistics (KNBS), approximately 1.7 million people lost their jobs due to the COVID-19 pandemic, which affected the informal job sector and caused the economy to slow (Ouma, Masai, and Nyadera 2020). Other national data indicate that two in three adults who lost all their income in 2020 were women. The most affected category was women working in the informal economy and dependent on daily wages (UN Kenya 2020). In addition to the economic shock experienced at household levels, social and mental well-being suffered. Various gender-based violence partners, the National Council of Administration of Justice, and the national domestic violence hotline reported a marked upsurge of sexual and gender-based violence occurrences (Bhalla 2020b, 2020a; Ngunjiri et al. 2020). Analysis of medical records also showed increases in sexual violence cases across outpatient departments in public health facilities in Kenya during the initial months of the pandemic (Barasa et al. 2021).

COVID-19 and its preventive measures caused devastating effects on the healthcare workforce, severely impacting the provision of healthcare services and reducing general health service availability. The healthcare workforce and infrastructure were diverted to serve the immediate needs of the outbreak (Barasa et al. 2021). Consequently, frontline workers at public health facilities were understaffed and ill equipped to manage COVID-19 cases in the hospitals, had limited COVID-19 training, and had limited access to personal protective equipment (PPE) (Ouma, Masai, and Nyadera 2020). All these factors contributed to significant service delivery disruptions and setbacks, including in the screening and treatment of major diseases such as HIV, tuberculosis, malaria, and cancer (Lagat et al. 2020). In response, the government provided additional funds for the recruitment of other health workers and the import of PPE (Barasa et al. 2021).

The literature has shown that in resource-limited settings, community health volunteers (CHVs) play a pivotal role in responding to major outbreaks, including disease surveillance and public health campaigns (Boyce and Katz 2019; Jaskiewicz and Tulenko 2012; WHO 2020). According to the Community Health Strategy of Kenya, CHVs are primarily responsible for health promotion, as well as preventive, curative and rehabilitation services at the community level (MoH 2020c). They implement health interventions that focus on building demand for existing health services, improving community awareness and health-seeking behaviors, providing health education, providing curative services for minor ailments, and giving referrals. Their efforts at the community level reduce the load on the already overburdened healthcare facilities. CHVs are also highly valued, as they can reach the most marginalized and vulnerable populations, including those in rural and informal settlements, through household visits. Women often participate as CHVs, despite being unpaid, for a combination of reasons including training opportunities, caring for the community in which they live, and wishing to participate in their own community's health advocacy and needs (Oliver et al. 2015).

From the onset of the COVID-19 pandemic, the MoH prioritized the deployment of CHVs to educate communities on COVID-19 prevention, treatment, and management to strengthen the home-based care option for patients with COVID-19 (MoH 2020b, 2020a). Additionally, CHVs were tasked with identification, contact tracing, and referral of identified assumptive COVID cases to isolation facilities. They also continued to provide essential healthcare services at the community and household levels.

In Kenya, most of those in the health and social sector workforce, including CHVs, are women (Kenya National Bureau of Statistics 2021). While women dominate the health sector, it is essential to note that the same women (and girls) are disproportionately affected by gender inequities and gendered power imbalances and face social risks at home, in the community, and in their places of work. These gendered inequities, social norms and practices intersect with CHVs' healthcare delivery role. Previous research shows that CHVs work in systems that tolerate and enable gendered vulnerabilities, affecting their life and work experiences (Raven et al. 2022). The pandemic period was no exception; during this time, gendered inequities and vulnerabilities were heightened, potentially having negative impacts on CHVs' experiences in their own households and during service delivery.

This chapter focuses on the experience of CHVs in implementing COVID-19 pandemic mitigation plans at the community and household level while maintaining their community health services. It explores CHVs' perceived needs and challenges, applying a gender-based lens to illuminate the intersection of the pandemic and the lives of CHVs as women in society and as service providers during the pandemic.

Methods and Process

In 2021, LVCT Health, a NGO based in Kenya, conducted a research study titled "Understanding and Mitigating Real-Time Differential Gendered Effects of the COVID-19 Outbreak: A Qualitative Study amongst Female Subpopulations within Nairobi and Migori Counties in Kenya." The study aimed to address critical questions surrounding the gendered vulnerabilities and impacts of the COVID-19 outbreak and response, as well as to identify opportunities for strengthening policies at both the county and national levels through enhanced gender analysis and mainstreaming. Given the limited gender analysis conducted during previous pandemics and the absence of real-time assessments, this project sought to fill significant gaps in both academic research and practical understanding of pandemic response.

The study employed an exploratory qualitative research design to investigate the perceptions and experiences of various populations, including CHVs, pregnant women/new mothers, female owners of small and medium-sized enterprises, adolescent girls, domestic workers, and policymakers. In-depth interviews were conducted with thirty-eight purposively sampled women CHVs: eighteen from Nairobi County's Kibera urban informal settlement and twenty drawn from rural Migori County. The interview guide focused on exploring the understanding of CHVs regarding the COVID-19 pandemic, the health-related challenges they face, the support they receive from their employers, and the difficulties they encounter while providing healthcare services during the pandemic. It included questions about CHVs' awareness of COVID-19, access to information, experiences in providing care during the pandemic, perceived risks due to COVID-19, government policies and responses, and the impact of COVID-19 on their daily lives and work. Open-ended questions explored the challenges and needs of CHVs during the COVID-19 pandemic, and the transcripts were analyzed through inductive coding (Elo and Kyngäs 2008).

Description of Participants and Study Setting

The study location was stratified by the identification of counties as either urban (Nairobi) or rural (Migori) (Kenya National Bureau of Statistics 2019). The rationale for stratification by rural versus urban is because of the differences between the two in terms of economic growth; access to water and sanitation services, health services, and social amenities; and the poverty index. They differ in their structural determinants of health, including COVID-19 pandemic response and recovery and other geographic inequities (Egede et al. 2017). The two counties bear characteristics that allowed for exploration of the gendered effects of COVID-19 among the selected target population. Within Nairobi, the study participant cohorts were selected from host communities in the urban informal settlements, specifically Kibera, while Migori was the township location. In Nairobi's urban informal settlements, residents often face economic challenges characterized by low incomes and limited access to formal employment opportunities. Many individuals in these areas rely on informal jobs to sustain their livelihoods. Access to healthcare services can be constrained due to financial barriers, inadequate infrastructure, and overcrowded facilities. Residents often experience higher rates of diseases and health issues due to poor sanitation and living conditions (Drummond et al. 2023). In contrast, in Migori rural areas, residents typically engage in agricultural activities as their primary source of income; the economy is largely based on subsistence farming, with limited access to formal employment opportunities. Healthcare services in rural areas are often scarce and distant, with inadequate infrastructure and healthcare professionals. Residents may face challenges accessing medical care due to geographical barriers and limited transportation options (Starnes et al. 2021). The sampled CHVs serve populations that often come from these economically disadvantaged backgrounds.

Various global and national reports and studies have described CHVs as "volunteer health workers," noting that they receive no salary, despite being proven to be a cost-effective way to extend health services to the hardest-to-reach communities (Nepomnyashchiy et al. 2020). The reports state that the problem of unpaid community health workers is widespread, with up to 60 percent of the volunteer health workers in low- and middle-income countries being affected (Nepomnyashchiy et al. 2020). In Kenya, the government mandated a monthly stipend of 2,000 Kenyan shillings (KES) (~US $20) for these individuals, yet the provision of this compensation remains primarily reliant on nongovernmental organizations and development partners (Abuya et al. 2021). Such support commonly takes the shape of transportation refunds, meal provisions, or a regular monthly payment, either fixed or contingent on performance (Abuya et al. 2021). Many of them face financial challenges due to their low or inconsistent pay, which may not be sufficient to meet their basic needs (Lusambili et al. 2021; Nyongesa, Onyango, and Kakai 2020). As a result, CHVs may struggle to support themselves and their families, facing difficulties in accessing healthcare services, education, and other essential resources. Despite these challenges, CHVs remain dedicated to their roles, driven by a strong sense of commitment to serving their communities and improving health outcomes.

Results

These findings shed light on various aspects related to the CHVs' understanding of the COVID-19 pandemic, their experiences in providing healthcare services during the pandemic, the support they receive, and the challenges they face. Through thematic analysis, the chapter delves into the key themes and insights derived from the responses provided by the CHVs during the interviews.

Description of Sample Size

The study analyzed demographic and occupational factors of CHVs sampled from the Migori and Nairobi regions, comprising twenty and eighteen participants respectively. A total of thirty-eight CHVs were surveyed, displaying a variety of characteristics indicative of their roles and experiences. The age of the CHVs ranged from twenty-eight to fifty-four years, with a median age of approximately forty-three years, suggesting a mature cohort with potentially extensive experience in community health.

In terms of marital status, a significant number of CHVs were married, which highlights the stability and community embeddedness essential for their roles, while the presence of widowed and single individuals might affect their availability and dedication to volunteer work. Family responsibilities were common among the CHVs, with the number of children ranging from none to seven. This diversity in family size implies varying commitments outside their roles, which could impact their availability for volunteering.

The CHVs demonstrated a broad spectrum of experience in their roles, spanning from less than a year to twenty-six years. This range highlights a dynamic mix of veteran insights and fresh perspectives within the group, which could be crucial for the effective transition of program responsibilities from donor to government support. Economically, many CHVs are involved in small businesses, such as farming and selling vegetables or operating niche markets like clothing and shoe sales, suggesting a high level of resourcefulness and strong connections within their communities. This entrepreneurial engagement underscores their ability to support themselves and contribute economically while fulfilling their roles as health volunteers.

Functionality of CHVs during the COVID-19 Pandemic

The CHVs recognized that they played a vital role in the community during COVID-19, viewing themselves as the "doctors in the community." CHVs acknowledged that they served the communities' interests, as they could attend to clients at the household level. As a result, the community accepted them as key players in the health sector during the pandemic. As the CHVs were from the communities they served, they felt that the community already had built-in trust toward them and considered them well-placed to conduct household visits and community sensitizations during the pandemic. They also appreciated the positive remarks by the MoH, whose officers were "really praising the CHVs saying that we are doing a great job in the community" (CHV, Nairobi).

Their roles in the COVID-19 pandemic response were clear to them—including case identification, referral of those suspected to have the virus, sensitization of the community on the preventive measures, monitoring of home-based care clients, and creating demand for vaccinations.

> First, I would refer them to go and get tested, give them information about not being in a gathered place, the importance of avoiding shaking of hands, sanitization, washing of hands and how they should cough and how they can cover their mouths while coughing. (CHV, Nairobi)

CHVs expressed that facility-based service providers relied on the CHVs' extensive knowledge to identify and refer COVID-19 cases at the community level, a task facility-based medics could not accomplish, as they did not make household and community visits. "We have a voice in the village because they understand. . . . They [facility-based medics and government] wait for a patient at the facility while some can't [go to the community]. It's a CHV to assist" (CHV, Nairobi).

CHVs led COVID-19-related public health talks and sensitization of community members on how to observe the COVID-19 preventive measures within households and the community. They developed information-sharing platforms using both in-person community gatherings and social media, such as WhatsApp groups. While most CHVs felt they received effective information on prevention and care from the MoH, they also felt it would have been helpful to receive more information beyond the preventive measures for COVID-19—such as information on the different strains of COVID-19 and their pathogenesis within individuals, the global context of the pandemic, and vaccine-related information.

Structural Challenges Faced by CHVs during the COVID-19 Response

The World Health Organization (WHO) has established critical foundational elements of successful CHV programs in resource-limited countries. These elements include providing training and supportive supervision to CHVs, a clear definition of their framework and roles within the healthcare system, adequate and appropriate incentives and compensation (monetary or in-kind), and sustained investments in their workforce (WHO 2017). However, data from the interviewed CHVs portrayed a different reality for those working on the ground.

All CHVs reported that they felt extremely vulnerable while conducting their activities in the community, as they did not have adequate access to PPE. They expressed fear of contracting the virus during household visits, in settings where the household members were on home-based care for COVID and were not using any protective equipment.

> We don't have protective equipment, especially when we are visiting these patients. We had wanted to be given masks and gloves because sometimes you can be forced to carry a patient. After all, they are not able to walk. It now forces us to touch them, yet we have not even been provided gloves. We have also not been provided with overalls so that we can wear to protect us from the disease. (CHV, Migori)

CHVs recognized it was the state's role to provide them with sanitizer, masks, and gloves, as they provided essential services in the community. Still, in almost all instances, civil society organizations provided any PPE that CHVs received. Others resorted to purchasing PPE using their own resources, an option they were unhappy about but felt helpless to rectify, as they prioritized their own and patients' safety. Some, however, had to continue to conduct their house visits without PPE and in constant fear of being infected.

> It is very easy for me to contract COVID as a result of my work because I have not really protected myself, and in case I find someone who has COVID because I am a CHV, it will force me to go and touch him and maybe take him to the hospital. You know that the sick person could now easily infect me with COVID-19, yes. (CHV, Nairobi)

CHVs working in Kiberia, the largest informal settlement in Nairobi, commented on the haphazard implementation of preventive measures. They remarked that there was a lack of consideration on how best to support the residents to adhere to these measures, given the poverty, environment and living conditions. For example, it was not possible, in informal urban settlements to maintain social distancing, as houses were close to each other. In other instances, lack of water meant no hand-washing stations in the home or community. In addition, almost all households CHVs visited did not have sanitizer or masks. Therefore, it was difficult to adhere to the public health policies, which heightened the risk of rapid community transmission.

> [The government] is doing a good job because it doesn't want people to suffer, but when giving these measures, it didn't think of how the normal citizen will earn a living. They just give measures and leave it at that, so you are forced to struggle, yet they keep collecting taxes. (CHV, Migori)

Beyond the provision of PPE, CHVs wished the government would cover their own medical bills and pay for the statutory National Health Insurance Fund due to the high likelihood they would contract the virus while conducting their duties. While most CHVs in Kibera were grateful that they had been prioritized to receive the vaccine free of charge, many of those in Migori could not access the vaccines, as distribution centers were far away and they could not afford the cost of transport.

In the early months of the COVID-19 outbreak, some CHVs were invited by their supervisors from the MoH to training sessions on COVID identification and prevention. In addition, local civil society organizations facilitated some pieces of training on the implementation of measures within communities. However, as the pandemic continued, CHVs remarked that they did not receive any other formal training on managing COVID-19, and some did not receive any training at all. Instead, almost all relied on the media's briefings to understand what was required of them as frontline workers and assumed roles without formal training. The inadequate training and supervision left them often unable to fully deliver on their mandate. In some instances, CHVs felt that the lack of training prevented them from providing clear information and quality care.

> Now, this vaccine that has come, we have not been explained very well about it. It is not clear about the vaccine. You find that people have different rumors about it. You even fear to go tell someone to go and get vaccinated. (CHV, Migori)

CHVs recommended that the frequency of training be increased, as information about COVID-19 was constantly evolving. They stated that their capacity development would lead to more proactive involvement in preventing the virus, and community members would value the information they shared.

Lack of stipend or remuneration Most CHVs in Kenya typically rely on remuneration and resources from not-for-profit organizations and agencies to offer community health services; the MoH does not compensate them monetarily. Almost all CHVs were acutely aware of their responsibility to provide healthcare during the pandemic. However, they remained frustrated by the lack of reimbursement, they felt they "try a lot to do community work, but you find that even something small, like a small stipend, we don't have" (CHV, Migori).

No CHV respondents had received any monetary incentives from the government. Aside from a salary, the lack of support for transport to households was a barrier to service provision.

> Again, sometimes you find that we lack means of transportation when you have a sick person in the community. Sometimes they stay a bit far from me, so you find it gets a bit late before I can't visit him because of the long distance. (CHV, Migori)

CHVs felt that being called "volunteers" denied them the opportunity to demand a stipend or performance-based incentives, yet they performed a critical service for the community's health interest. They also stated that although they voiced their needs, there was no response from the government on how their lack of compensation affected their performance. "But when it comes to giving us a stipend that will motivate us to do the work itself, it has never been sorted out from up there" (CHV, Migori).

Some had to abandon their health care service provision due to lack of renumeration, even in the middle of the pandemic, and opted for other commitments that brought them some income for survival. Others felt they still had an obligation to deliver services at the community level: "So you just bite your tongue and do the work saying that God will pay you." (CHV, Nairobi).

In the context of COVID-19 and the resulting increased economic insecurity and reduced access to necessities, some remarked that they expected the Ministry of Health (MoH) to support them in meeting domestic needs by providing in-kind goods, such as food vouchers. Overall, they sought some sort of recognition for the sacrifices they were making and the services they were providing despite the challenging environment and continuous exposure to COVID-19 during household visits. However, this recognition was not forthcoming, making them more disgruntled.

> No, there's no support. There's even this one day I was asking, how is it that we are the ones who work in the community down there so that the government knows what's happening down there. I even walk through sewerage in my community to get to my area to give a report to our bosses so that they can hand it in. You have to give them the report so they can also hand it in. We are the ones who are down there in the slums. So we know what is happening. So I was asking myself, we should be called and told, "Take these vouchers, go do some shopping or do this and that with it." I don't get any support. (CHV, Nairobi)

In some instances, CHVs reported that they were running micro- and small-scale businesses, in addition to their CHV roles, that would earn them an income to sustain themselves. Businesses included selling second-hand clothes (*mitumba*), running a hair salon, and selling food in the market and in restaurants. Some CHVs admitted that they preferred committing time toward their businesses, as they could earn a living from it to sustain their families, unlike risking their lives for voluntary work that did not reward them monetarily.

> We used to conduct a business. CHV work is volunteer work. A project has to come, and they say they will support us with this or that. So we used to conduct business. My business actually went down. (CHV, Migori)

These double shifts (CHV health promotion work and business) affected their performance at work, as well as making it challenging to deliver vital community health services effectively.

Lack of integration into the national MoH service delivery registry Almost all CHVs we interviewed felt disgruntled by the lack of recognition by MoH and the government did not feel that they were treated like professionals.

> They should put strategies and recognize CHV is on the ground and are more informed on what's happening there. They should consider us as part of the government as well because we work with them, but (they/MoH) don't recognize us as part of them; they view us as community members only. (CHV, Nairobi)

The CHVs felt they sacrificed their lives and livelihoods by voluntarily leading the COVID-19 prevention initiatives at the community level with limited or no government support, and "the work we do is recommendable" (CHV, Nairobi).

They stated that they were fully aware of the difficulties in implementing the stipulated COVID-19 prevention measures and providing essential services during the pandemic. Despite this, MoH did not address their concerns.

> CHVs are the people on the ground. We share our experiences, but we are not heard. We tell them [government/MoH] about the experiences, but they do nothing except to do what is good for the country instead of coming to the ground and see what is happening. (CHV, Nairobi)

Some implied their role was more critical than facility-based service providers. They felt "it's us who first identify the patients before the clinicians . . . because we are the ones who go round interacting with people to see how they are keeping on" (CHV, Nairobi).

But they still lacked the needed recognition or support by the government. They did not have a voice, and the government did not respond when they explained their predicaments. "Yeah, it's us who have a voice, but our voice is never heard. We have a voice because it's us who first identify the patients before the clinicians, but we are forgotten as CHVs" (CHV, Nairobi).

Narratives by the CHVs illustrated how they remain poorly integrated into existing health systems, which contributed to fragmentation in health care delivery from community to facility. They proposed that the government could ensure that they were included on the MoH payroll as salaried workers and be accredited in national MoH registries, indicating that their efforts and needs were being addressed. They felt this would be the only way they could be meaningfully engaged in decision-making and well represented in work planning and the only way they could advocate for providing much-needed resources.

Hostile reception by community members CHVs experienced difficulties as they carried out the community-level campaign for COVID-19. They were constantly suspected of carrying the virus as they made household visits and were thus seen as likely to infect others. CHVs also reported that community members were reluctant to engage with them, as they were labeled as being responsible for committing community members to isolation and quarantine if they were found to have COVID-19-like symptoms. As a result, the community grew skeptical of CHVs. During household visits, CHVs received hostile remarks or were ignored when they emphasized the need for household members to follow COVID-19 preventive measures such as social distancing, self-isolation, or wearing masks.

> When it comes to experience, there is nothing good I have seen. It has been very difficult for me. Things have changed because you can't go to households now. We used to go before, being very free. So now, when you go to visit people in their households, you can't sit very near to that person because you don't know who has COVID and who doesn't. They also don't trust me. . . . You even fear going somewhere. You can't even go to knock at someone's household for help. They won't even open the door for you. (CHV, Nairobi)

The community also had high expectations from CHVs beyond providing health services. In many instances, the CHVs reported that the community members expected aid such as food from them, a provision the CHVs could not offer. This was mainly in the most vulnerable households, such as

> those who are very, very poor that think that when you go to talk to them, there is some aid that you are taking to them, yet there is no such aid. You can't even go to ask someone how they have woken up, whether they have gone to the clinic. They will ask you, "Did you bring me food?" (CHV, Nairobi)

Additionally, the lack of recognition by the government for CHVs as formal service providers at the community level contributed to the rejection by community members.

> Because the people don't respect us because we have not received training from the government, they have not accepted us since some we live with them in the same community and question us, for example, when did we go to college. (CHV, Nairobi)

The interlinking dynamics of community members' fear of COVID and isolation with CHVs' lack of renumeration and recognition affected the performance of CHVs during the COVID-19 pandemic.

The Gendered Perspective of Community Health Service Delivery

Competing demand from increased unpaid household burden and childcare

Typically, in the Kenyan context, childcare is the responsibility of mothers. CHVs noted that even though their spouses were at home due to COVID-19 response measures, the women still exclusively bore the burden of childcare and food provision.

> You find that women are the ones who take care of children more than men when men come from work they go sit in groups with people they don't know if they have COVID then come home demanding for food or start fighting the wife and children. So this disease has come to separate families because the wife feels like they have a huge burden. So it's a challenge to everyone. (CHV, Nairobi)

Almost all acknowledged that it was their responsibility to pay school fees for their children, ensure all meals were provided, and attend to their school-going children at home due to school closures. With schools closed due to COVID-19, they were responsible for the children at home, with limited income, which caused great anxiety.

> The second thing, my children will be affected even more. They don't go to school, and they don't read. They are just in the house. It's hard to get food to eat, so it is a challenge that also affects children mentally. It will therefore continue to negatively impact my life. (CHV, Migori)

The increased violence against adolescent girls and boys exacerbated their fears, as mothers felt their children were increasingly at risk.

> It has really affected me in that my children do not go to school as they should, there are a lot of pregnancies because of them staying at home, and there is a lot of intimate partner violence in my village, and I am forced to go to them and maybe have a talk with them. (CHV, Migori)

CHVs' care burden also included extended family, as CHVs felt that "family will be affected because you can no longer assist your mother upcountry. It affects all corners" (CHV, Nairobi).

Despite the increased unpaid homecare, all the CHVs admitted that they received no support from their employer (the government). They did not receive any parental or childcare leave to look after their family and were expected to work continuously. They also did not receive any pay or sick leave when they fell ill and could not look after their family or work.

> We don't get any form of leave like personally, I have been sick, but still my employer insists that they need reports from me, so it forces me to delegate my work to another CHV so as to go to my village and pick reports for me. (CHV, Nairobi)

Increased Risk of Infection to Family and Household Members

Most CHVs stated that they had to visit over a hundred households during the pandemic period. They felt this exposure increased their risk of contracting the virus, as most homes did not have access to sanitizers, soap, water, or masks. As mothers, the women CHVs constantly feared infecting their children and spouses with COVID-19 due to their exposure at work.

> You see, in my family, I have my husband and children. Let's say I am coming back home from somewhere. Where I am from, I don't know whether I might have come into contact with someone who has the COVID virus. I come with that at home. You see, now I have spread it to my whole family because we are all together in the house. Yeah, because you can't stay apart when you are one family. So you just stay in close proximity to each other, yet you don't know. (CHV, Nairobi)

They felt the government should prioritize PPE distribution and vaccination to CHVs with families and their household members to minimize these risks. Yet the CHVs had limited access to vaccines. They observed vaccine provision inequities by the MoH:

> It's possible because as things are, there are no preventive measures at all, be it vaccination, PPEs? Because of this lockdown, the vaccine should be availed to us to help protect our people. We just hear it's given to the big people while down here. We are just using masks, hand washing and observing social distance, and we have not been immunized. We must be worried. (CHV, Nairobi)

CHVs explained that while some of them had received the first dose, most had challenges making appointments for the second. Vaccine distribution centers were often far from their locality, and there was no transport reimbursement, or they arrived at distribution centers to find that there were no vaccines in stock. One CHV was told she must get a group of at least eight workers together for the vaccine team to visit her village, but it was challenging to coordinate everyone's schedule to accommodate one time. While the government stated that frontline healthcare providers would be prioritized for the vaccine, CHVs' ambiguous status meant it was not clear if they qualified. Yet CHVs understood why they should be given priority in vaccination given their nature of work—visiting households where people may be ill, which increased their likelihood of acquiring and transmitting the virus.

A shift in gender norms at the household level Ordinarily, in the Kenyan patriarchal system, men are the income earners. But due to the job losses occasioned by the pandemic, this responsibility was assumed by the CHVs. They felt this responsibility was huge, given that they did not receive any monetary remuneration from the government. Some of the burden, particularly the economic burden experienced, was due to a shift in decision-making and income generation. For some CHVs, their spouse was ordinarily the primary breadwinner. However, their spouses passed on this responsibility to CHVs, who did not earn a stipend under current circumstances. Nonetheless, "the women are the ones who are left with the workload" (CHV, Nairobi).

This meant that they took on extra work and additional jobs to try to provide for the family, thus overburdening themselves.

> When I found out that my husband had lost his job, I remained as the person to provide in the house. I found a lot of difficulties. To date, I do find it difficult because I am forced to do more than I used to. Even if I get money from the mentorship, it is still not enough, so I am forced to sell vegetables. I sew things like masks that can give me money apart from my other work that I was doing. It forced me to know how to plait such that I try and find money and bring to the house for people to eat. (CHV, Migori)

Experience of gender-based violence and risk to personal safety CHVs were cognizant of the increased vulnerabilities women faced in the communities during the pandemic. They attributed the increased occurrence of gender-based violence to poverty, loss of livelihoods, lack of necessities such as food in the house, and use of alcohol as a coping strategy, which increased tension and conflict between spouses.

> Like this pandemic has affected most of us, especially women. Like by that time, the husband has left to fend same to the mother in the household. But now it is time. . . . No one is leaving the house. Everyone is in the house, and the person who suffers is the woman. Sometimes you were used to asking 20 for food and that point in time when you ask from them 20 you'll be insulted maybe physically violated. (CHV, Nairobi)

CHVs who experienced violence shared that this was often due to requesting funds from their spouse in order to access necessities. Even as health service providers were responding to cases of gender-based violence in the community, they were not exempt from being at risk or experiencing violence within their households, much like other women in the community.

> It will have affected me greatly in my life because it is breaking my home. When I sit with my husband in the house during this COVID period, and there is no money when I try and ask him for food or something, it becomes a fight then he leaves and doesn't come back, it is only him who knows where he goes. (CHV, Nairobi)

Negative mental health status and limited social support CHVs reported feeling isolated, anxious, and ostracized during the pandemic. The uncertainty about the spread of the pandemic and the devastation each new wave would cause was overwhelming. Social distancing and isolation contributed to their negative mental health status. In addition, unrewarded efforts to generate income and provide for their families increased their distress.

> Yes, you can lack some things that can even make you want to commit suicide so that you are not bothered with all these troubles. The money is scarce, there is not enough food, and school fees are also lacking. (CHV, Nairobi)

Additionally, they constantly feared contracting the disease from household members during visits.

> So you get to worry; I have a life to live, I have a family which I live with. I have to protect my family by protecting myself in that I don't expose myself and take corona to them. So sometimes, it affects me mentally because I know I have interacted with possibly corona-positive cases. So it's a challenge. (CHV, Nairobi)

The increased insecurity in their neighborhoods and work-related trauma from handling critical patients and deceased COVID-19 patients brought on mental health anguish. In addition, some CHVs felt helpless, as the government did not help them to support the ailing community members as much as they wished to, which led to low morale. Community members had high expectations of food and material support from CHVs, which was impossible to provide.

Most CHVs were unable to seek psychosocial support due to lack of funds for the available paid mental health services or due to social distancing, lockdown, and curfews, and some feared exposing themselves to the virus more than necessary. Some CHVs were able to reach out to their friends and family for debriefing to relieve their stress, and a lucky few were able to access psychological support programs provided by civil society organizations.

Discussion

The COVID-19 pandemic caused significant disruption in providing healthcare services to communities. It increased vulnerabilities, significantly affecting the lives of marginalized populations such as those living in informal urban settlements and rural areas. These populations could not access health services related to sexual and reproductive health, immunization, maternal health, and post-violence care. In addition, the community was ill informed and reluctant to seek COVID-19 clinical care or adopt prevention measures. In its effort to disrupt COVID-19 community transmission and ensure the continuity of essential health services, the government tasked CHVs to act as frontline workers in the community. CHVs conducted disease surveillance, provided referrals, made linkages with health facilities and isolation centers, and monitored home-based care clients. They were responsible for community awareness regarding COVID-19 risk factors, symptoms, and preventive measures, as well as for dispelling myths and misconceptions among community members. CHVs felt competent to fulfill this role, as they resided in the communities, were well accepted in most instances, and could reach the most vulnerable with services because they understood their plight in the community they served and lived in.

However, gender roles and norms structured the experiences of CHVs, restricting their ability to provide efficient healthcare and negatively impacting their well-being. CHVs found it hard to balance their voluntary role in health delivery against homecare and income-generating activities to survive the pandemic and sustain their families. Consequently, they experienced mental health challenges due to burnout, which was layered onto work-related trauma and fear of transmitting COVID to their families. Like other women in their communities, they experienced increased gender-based violence. Most did not have access to psychosocial support, alternative homecare arrangements for their families, or sources of additional income when household finances were affected by the pandemic. The MoH produced COVID-19 response guidelines for frontline health workers that were completely gender-blind, and their implementation did not serve the unique needs of women CHVs. CHVs remained unpaid, with no formal voice in the pandemic response to which they were essential. They were made increasingly vulnerable during the pandemic and still expected to deliver services optimally.

Consequently, CHVs also felt ill equipped to manage the COVID cases in the community and provide other essential routine health services. Due to limited resources, they visited fewer households, restricted their data reporting on different components of health other than COVID-19, and resisted offering referrals to community members due to hostile reception. Additionally, there was a shift in the services offered during the pandemic. CHVs assumed COVID-19 prevention service delivery and dropped their routine care. These changes in healthcare service delivery may lead to adverse long-term health outcomes and poorer well-being within the population.

There is a demonstrated need to invest in community health systems—from the CHV workforce itself to resources to help them be functional and effective in health promotion, prevention, and pandemic response. Policymakers and health system managers also need to clearly define CHVs' responsibilities with respect to the provision of non-pandemic-related but equally essential vital health services amid a crisis.

Recommendations for Gender-Specific Policy Enhancements

Given the multifaceted challenges faced by CHVs, particularly during health emergencies like the COVID-19 pandemic, there is a pressing need for policies that are not only gender-sensitive but also equity-informed. Such policies should acknowledge and address the diverse realities of CHVs, considering factors such as socioeconomic status, cultural background, and geographic disparities in addition to gender:

- **Comprehensive policymaking participation:** Female CHVs should have significant representation in policymaking processes to ensure that their insights and experiences directly inform health strategies and interventions. To enhance the gender-specific approach in the rollout of policies to address the challenges faced by CHVs during the COVID-19 pandemic, it is important to consider the unique gendered impacts observed. Further, and beyond gender, we need to broaden participation to include CHVs from diverse backgrounds. This includes not only women but also representatives from minority ethnic groups, various socioeconomic backgrounds, and different geographical regions. Such inclusive representation ensures that policies are crafted from a wide range of perspectives, which can enhance the relevance and effectiveness of health strategies and interventions.
- **Integration of multidimensional gender analysis:** Ensure that gender analysis is a foundational aspect of policy development. This involves assessing the different impacts of health emergencies on men and women and recognizing the increased vulnerabilities that women face, especially those in health service roles like CHVs. This analysis should inform all aspects of policy planning, ensuring that measures are sensitive to the needs of all genders.
- **Holistic approach to addressing gender-based violence:** Policies should directly address the surge in gender-based violence, which often increases during health crises. Alongside gender-based violence, policies should also address other forms of discrimination and violence that may affect CHVs based on other aspects of their identity. This includes racial discrimination or violence based on disability, ensuring that comprehensive support mechanisms are in place and ensuring that health responses integrate services for survivors of violence.
- **Support structures for CHVs:** Recognizing the dual burden carried by female CHVs, policies should include provisions for support structures like childcare, flexible working hours, and mental health services. These support systems can help mitigate the burden of unpaid care work that predominantly falls on women.
- **Economic support for female CHVs:** Given the economic challenges highlighted in this chapter, particularly for women, policies could propose specific stipends or financial incentives for female CHVs. This approach

acknowledges their critical role and compensates for the lack of formal payment structures, which can be particularly impactful for women, who are often in economically precarious positions.

- **Training and capacity building:** Implement training programs that are not only accessible but also tailored to address the needs of female CHVs, focusing on empowerment, leadership, and specific health service delivery in crises. These programs should aim to strengthen their capacities to manage health services effectively while also addressing any gender-specific health needs of the community.
- **Strengthening participation in policymaking:** Encourage and facilitate the involvement of female CHVs in the decision-making process. This can be achieved by establishing advisory panels or committees that include significant representation of women, particularly those from the community health sectors, to ensure that their experiences and insights inform policy responses.

By adopting these intersectional strategies, policies will be better positioned to support all CHVs comprehensively, ensuring that responses to health emergencies are not only gender-sensitive but also attuned to the diverse realities of socioeconomic status, ethnicity, and other critical factors. This approach ensures that policy development and health system responses are effectively aligned with the needs of every community member, promoting outcomes that are both equitable and effective across all demographics.

Conclusion

Like so many women healthcare workers around the world, CHVs filled an essential service role during Kenya's COVID-19 response, providing information and care in hard-to-reach communities. However, again like so many feminized healthcare roles, this essential labor was not valued through the provision of a salary or even adequate PPE. Meanwhile CHVs faced the same challenges as many other women during the pandemic—trying to manage both increased paid and unpaid care responsibilities and protect themselves and their children from increased violence. CHVs, particularly those from economically marginalized communities and working within the informal economy, also grappled with the precariousness of informal work that offered little security in times of crisis. The intersection of gender with socioeconomic disadvantages meant that these women were disproportionately affected by the pandemic, struggling to protect themselves and their families from heightened violence and economic instability. Their perseverance throughout the crisis is justification that their demands for fair working conditions, access to healthcare for themselves, adequate supplies to care for others, and better support systems be heeded, underscoring the urgent need for comprehensive policy reforms. Recognizing the layered challenges faced by CHVs justifies the need for a health system that is responsive not only to gender but also to the economic realities that shape their experiences and capacities to respond to health emergencies.

References

Abuya, Timothy, Daniel Mwanga, Melvin Obadha, Charity Ndwiga, George Odwe, Daniel Kavoo, John Wanyugu, Charlotte Warren, and Smisha Agarwal. 2021. "Incentive Preferences for Community Health Volunteers in Kenya: Findings from a Discrete Choice Experiment." *BMJ Open* 11 (7): e048059.

Aluga, Martin A. 2020. "Coronavirus Disease 2019 (COVID-19) in Kenya: Preparedness, Response and Transmissibility." *Journal of Microbiology, Immunology, and Infection* 53 (5): 671–673. https://doi.org/10.1016/j.jmii.2020.04.011.

Barasa, Edwine, Jacob Kazungu, Stacey Orangi, Evelyn Kabia, Morris Ogero, and Kadondi Kasera. 2021. "Indirect Health Effects of the COVID-19 Pandemic in Kenya: A Mixed Methods Assessment." *BMC Health Services Research* 21 (1). https://doi.org/10.1186/s12913-021-06726-4.

Bhalla, Nita. 2020a. "Futures Destroyed: COVID-19 Unleashes 'Shadow Pandemics' on Africa's Girls." Thomas Reuters Foundation News, August 20. https://news.trust.org/item/20200820135640-yl2ii/.

Bhalla, Nita. 2020b. "Kenya Orders Probe into Rise in Violence against Women and Girls during Pandemic." *Reuters*, July 6. https://www.reuters.com/article/us-health-coronavirus-kenya-women-trfn/kenya-orders-probe-into-rise-in-violence-against-women-and-girls-during-pandemic-idUSKBN2472ER.

Boyce, Matthew R., and Rebecca Katz. 2019. "Community Health Workers and Pandemic Preparedness: Current and Prospective Roles." *Frontiers in Public Health* 26 (7): 62. https://doi.org/10.3389/fpubh.2019.00062.

Drummond, John Amin, Bruce D. Malamud, Joe Mulligan, Vera Bukachi, Manshur Talib, Amos Wandera, Mark Pelling, and Faith E. Taylor. 2023. "COVID-19 Interventions in an Informal Settlement: A Spatial Analysis of Accessibility in Kibera, Kenya."

Journal of Transport Geography 113: 103704. https://www.sciencedirect.com/science/article/pii/S096669232300176X.

Egede, Leonard E., Delia Voronca, Rebekah J. Walker, and Craig Thomas. 2017. "Rural-Urban Differences in Trends in the Wealth Index in Kenya: 1993–2009." *Annals of Global Health* 83 (2): 248–258.

Elo, Satu, and Helvi Kyngäs. 2008. "The Qualitative Content Analysis Process." *Journal of Advanced Nursing* 62 (1): 107–115. https://doi.org/10.1111/j.1365-2648.2007.04569.x.

Jaskiewicz, Wanda, and Kate Tulenko. 2012. "Increasing Community Health Worker Productivity and Effectiveness: A Review of the Influence of the Work Environment." *Human Resources for Health* 10 (1): 1–9.

Kenya National Bureau of Statistics. 2019. "Volume I: Population by County and Sub-County." In *2019 Kenya Population and Housing Census*, 1–38. Nairobi: Kenya National Bureau of Statistics. https://housingfinanceafrica.org/app/uploads/VOLUME-I-KPHC-2019.pdf.

Kenya National Bureau of Statistics. 2021. *Economic Survey 2021*. Nairobi: Kenya National Bureau of Statistics. https://www.knbs.or.ke/wp-content/uploads/2021/09/Economic-Survey-2021.pdf.

Lagat, Harison, Monisha Sharma, Edward Kariithi, George Otieno, David Katz, Sarah Masyuko, Mary Mugambi, Beatrice Wamuti, Bryan Weiner, and Carey Farquhar. 2020. "Impact of the COVID-19 Pandemic on HIV Testing and Assisted Partner Notification Services, Western Kenya." *AIDS and Behavior* 24 (11): 3010–3013. https://doi.org/10.1007/s10461-020-02938-7.

Lusambili, Adelaide M., Njeri Nyanja, Sophie Vusha Chabeda, Marleen Temmerman, Lucy Nyaga, Jerim Obure, and Anthony Ngugi. 2021. "Community Health Volunteers Challenges and Preferred Income Generating Activities for Sustainability: A Qualitative Case Study of Rural Kilifi, Kenya." *BMC Health Services Research* 21: 1–9.

Ministry of Health. 2020a. "COVID-19 Campaign Posters." Nairobi: Kenya Ministry of Health.

Ministry of Health. 2020b. "COVID 19 Protocols and Guidelines." Nairobi: Kenya Ministry of Health.

Ministry of Health. 2020c. "Kenya Community Health Strategy 2020–2025." Nairobi: Kenya Ministry of Health.

Mueller, Valerie, Karen A. Grépin, Atonu Rabbani, Bianca Navia, Anne S. W. Ngunjiri, and Nicole Wu. 2022. "Food Insecurity and COVID-19 Risk in Low- and Middle-Income Countries." *Applied Economic Perspectives and Policy* 44 (1): 92–109. https://doi.org/https://doi.org/10.1002/aepp.13200.

Mueller, Valerie, Anne Ngunjiri, Atonu Rabbani, Heang Tan, Nicole Wu, and Karen Grépin. 2022. "COVID-19 Impacts on Women's Well-Being: Insights from a Longitudinal Study in Kenya." *Gender & COVID-19 Project.* https://www.genderandcovid-19.org/wp-content/uploads/2022/06/PAC00529_Gender-Covid-19-brief-from-Kenya-002.pdf.

Nepomnyashchiy, Lyudmila, Carey Westgate, Ashley Wang, Helen Olsen, Prashant Yadav, and Madeleine Ballard. 2020. "Protecting Community Health Workers: PPE Needs and Recommendations for Policy Action." https://www.cgdev.org/publication/protecting-community-health-workers-ppe-needs-and-recommendations-policy-action.

Ngunjiri, Anne, Lilian Otiso, Anthony Mwaniki, Carol Omondi, and Jane Thiomi. 2020. "Violence Against Women and Girls amidst COVID-19 Pandemic: LVCT Health Experience." Nairobi: LVCT Health.

Nyongesa, Mureka B., Rosebella O. Onyango, and Rose Kakai. 2020. "The Role of Income Generating Activities in Sustainable Retention of Community Health Volunteers in Primary Health-Care Service Provision in Bungoma County, Kenya." *Annals of Community Health* 8: 2–13.

Oliver M., A. Geniets, N. Winters, I. Rega, and S. Mbae. 2015. "What Do Community Health Workers Have to Say about Their Work, and How Can This Inform Improved Programme Design? A Case Study with CHWs within Kenya." *Global Health Action* 8(1): 27168. https://doi.org/10.3402/gha.v8.27168.

Ouma, Polet N., Abednego N. Masai, and Israel N. Nyadera. 2020. "Health Coverage and What Kenya Can Learn from the COVID-19 Pandemic." *Journal of Global Health* 10 (2): 020362. https://doi.org/10.7189/jogh.10.020362.

Oyando, Robinson, Stacey Orangi, Daniel Mwanga, Jessie Pinchoff, Timothy Abuya, Eva Muluve, Faith Mbushi, Karen Austrian, and Edwine Barasa. 2021. "Assessing Equity and the Determinants of Socio-Economic Impacts of COVID-19: Results from a Cross-Sectional Survey in Three Counties in Kenya." *Wellcome Open Research* 6: 339. https://doi.org/10.12688/wellcomeopenres.17367.1.

Pinchoff, Jessie, Karen Austrian, Nandita Rajshekhar, Timothy Abuya, Beth Kangwana, Rhoune Ochako, James Benjamin Tidwell, et al. 2021. "Gendered Economic, Social and Health Effects of the COVID-19 Pandemic and Mitigation Policies in Kenya: Evidence from a Prospective Cohort Survey in Nairobi Informal Settlements." *BMJ Open* 11 (3): e042749. https://doi.org/10.1136/bmjopen-2020-042749.

Raven, Joanna, Haja Wurie, Amuda Baba, Abdulai Jawo Bah, Laura Dean, Kate Hawkins, Ayesha Idriss, et al. 2022. "Supporting Community Health Workers in Fragile Settings from a Gender Perspective: A Qualitative Study." *BMJ Open* 12 (2): e052577. https://doi.org/10.1136/bmjopen-2021-052577.

Starnes, Joseph R., Jane Wamae, Vincent Okoth, Daniele J. Ressler, Vincent Were, Lawrence P. O. Were, Troy D. Moon, and Richard Wamai. 2021. "Population-Based Socio-Demographic Household Assessment of Livelihoods and Health among Communities in Migori County, Kenya over Multiple Timepoints (2021, 2024, 2027): A Study Protocol." *PLoS One* 16 (8): e0256555.

UN Kenya. 2020. "Covid-19 Gender Assessment: Gender Perspective (Kenya)." UN Women. https://data.unwomen.org/sites/default/files/documents/Publications/COVID-19%20Gender%20Assessment_Kenya.pdf.

Wangari, Edwin N., Peter Gichuki, Angelyne A. Abuor, Jacqueline Wambui, Stephen O. Okeyo, Henry T. N. Oyatsi, Shadrack Odikara, and Benard W. Kulohoma. 2021. "Kenya's Response to the COVID-19 Pandemic: A Balance between Minimising Morbidity and Adverse Economic Impact." *AAS Open Research* 4 (3). https://doi.org/10.12688/aasopenres.13156.2.

WHO. 2017. *Community Health Worker Programmes in the WHO Africa Region: Evidence and Options Policy Brief.* Geneva: World Health Organization.

WHO. 2020. "What Do We Know about Community Health Workers? A Systematic Review of Existing Reviews." *Human Resources for Health Observer Series: 19*. Geneva: World Health Organization.

World Bank Group. 2021. *Socioeconomic Impacts of COVID-19 in Kenya on Households: Rapid Response Phone Survey Round 1*. Washington DC: World Bank Group. https://openknowledge.worldbank.org/bitstream/handle/10986/35173/Socioeconomic-Impacts-of-COVID-19-in-Kenya-on-Households-Rapid-Response-Phone-Survey-Round-One.pdf?sequence=6&isAllowed=y.

8 "We the Women Do a Lot of Support": Experiences of Women Market Traders, Women Living in Slums, and Women with Disabilities in Lagos, Nigeria, during the COVID-19 Pandemic

Amy Oyekunle, Uche Ralph-Opara, Patience Agada, and Oluwakemi Odukoya

Introduction

In Nigeria, the first case of COVID-19 was reported on February 27, 2020. Just three months later, the number of cases had surpassed 10,000, with 287 confirmed deaths. Lagos State remained the epicenter of the outbreak (Abayomi et al. 2024). From April 1, 2020, the Nigerian government directed all residents to stay indoors with imposed curfews from dusk to dawn across several states and the closure of religious institutions. All international airports and land borders were closed for a month, including a ban on interstate travel (Federal Government of Nigeria 2020). On May 18, 2020, the Nigerian Federal Government released the National COVID-19 Pandemic Multi-Sectoral Response Plan (the Plan), which focused on preventing, containing, and mitigating COVID-19 infections as well as addressing the socioeconomic impacts of the pandemic through the provision of palliatives or aid. President Muhammed Buhari later signed the 2021 COVID-19 health protection regulation, a forty-two-item list with guidance on the restriction of gatherings, offenses, mandatory treatment, and enforcement of the regulations (Dan-Nwafor et al. 2020; President, Federal Republic of Nigeria 2021). The Plan included implementing nationwide nonpharmaceutical measures such as the use of face masks, hand washing and hand sanitizing, the cessation of nonessential movements, and social distancing (President, Federal Republic of Nigeria 2021). People were confined to their homes and unable to perform their usual income-generating activities, resulting in significant economic and social costs, such as increased poverty, crime, substance use, and domestic violence, with effects being most pronounced for women and marginalized populations, especially those living in poverty (United Nations

Nigeria 2020). The Federal Government attempted to cushion the effect of these socioeconomic impacts by providing support in the form of cash transfers, food aid, and personal protective equipment to vulnerable households.

In this chapter, we explore how women who are informal traders, who live in slums, and who have disabilities experienced lockdown. We selected these groups of women as being among those made marginalized by prepandemic economic and social structures. Moreover, such constituent groups contribute to broader considerations throughout the chapters in this volume, demonstrating the diverse intersectional experiences of women during COVID-19. We ask how the pandemic affected these diverse women and girls, particularly in relation to their unpaid work and risks of sexual and gender-based violence (SGBV). We found, common to the broader narrative in this edition, that the experiences of the Nigerian women we interviewed involving financial insecurity, increased unpaid care work, and physical insecurity reflected not only the lack of gender considerations within the pandemic response but also their social locations at the intersections of multiple inequities.

Gender and the Nigerian Woman

In Nigeria, religious and cultural norms entrenched in patriarchal values inform practices and behavior. As a result, discriminatory laws and policies, poverty, corruption, and a lack of accountability for gender-related commitments often disproportionately affect women and girls. The British Council's report on gender in Nigeria states that Nigerian women and girls have significantly worse life opportunities than men, as well as women, in comparable societies (Chimhowu, Zeitlyn, and Dada 2012). Violence compounds and reinforces this disadvantage (World Bank 2022; Chimhowu, Zeitlyn, and Dada 2012). The report also finds that Nigeria's National Gender Policy has yet to bear fruit and notes that the implementation of the Convention on the Elimination of all Forms of Discrimination against Women (CEDAW) has stalled in Nigeria (Chimhowu, Zeitlyn, and Dada 2012). One in three Nigerian women and girls age fifteen to twenty-four has been a victim of violence (Chimhowu, Zeitlyn, and Dada 2012; NPC and ICF 2019). In Nigeria, violence against women is deeply rooted in cultural beliefs in the society at large. Gender differences are often created and sustained through societal and traditional customs, conventions, norms, and regulations (Chimhowu, Zeitlyn, and Dada 2012).

In the presence of these enabling factors, the COVID-19 pandemic and its associated policy measures led to a surge in the number of cases of domestic violence reported by women. The Lagos State Domestic and Sexual Violence Response Team reported a threefold increase in the number of telephone calls received through their hotlines in one month (Chimhowu, Zeitlyn, and Dada 2012). These were primarily due to spouses having to stay together for prolonged periods and the absence of getaways such as work or other activities outside the home environment (Chimhowu, Zeitlyn, and Dada 2012).

Nigeria ranks 139 out of 149 countries on the World Economic Forum's Gender Gap Index, and civil society groups have raised concerns that the country may be regressing in terms of women's representation in leadership (UNICEF Nigeria n.d.; World Economic Forum 2021). Only seven female senators (7.63 percent) and twenty representatives (5.56 percent) were elected in 2015 as opposed to nine senators and twenty-five representatives in 2007 (IPU Parline n.d.). This is below the global average and well behind South Africa and Rwanda. Nigeria's House of Representatives has 360 members; of these, only 22 are women (CLGF 2019). While the Nigerian constitution provides for gender equality and nondiscrimination, women continue to suffer injustices and marginalization. In Nigeria, women are often excluded from decision-making at all levels by male-dominated patronage networks, the absence of agreed-upon quotas, and a party system that fails to nominate women candidates for electable seats. Fear of violence and restrictions on mobility may also deter women in some instances. Current patterns will likely continue unless women are represented in elected bodies where major spending decisions are made (IPU Parline n.d.; CLGF 2019).

In Nigeria, women compose the majority of informal-sector workers. A 2018 estimate by the International Labor Organization shows that 93 percent of all employment in Nigeria is informal, with 95 percent of women working in the informal sector, compared to 90 percent of men (UNDP 2020). Though many women are involved in subsistence agriculture and off-farm activities, men are five times more likely than women to own land. Women own only 10 percent of the land in Nigeria despite being responsible for 70 to 80 percent of agricultural labor in the country (FAO n.d.). Land ownership and land tenure give women security and provide them with the key to access other resources and opportunities. The economic gap between men and women in Nigeria is largely influenced by educational disparities, the poor political representation of women, and cultural norms. Gender differences amplify this gap when women do not have the financial capability to access healthcare services adequately and are therefore more likely to suffer poor health outcomes.

Before the COVID-19 pandemic, women with disabilities already faced a doubling of discrimination as women and as people with disabilities. They had poor access to healthcare, including sexual and reproductive health, higher risks of SGBV, higher unemployment rates, and limited inclusion in leadership and decision-making platforms and opportunities. Furthermore, women with disabilities were more likely to be institutionalized and experience inequality in hiring, promotion rates and pay for equal work, access to training and retraining, and access to credit and other productive sources, and they rarely participated in economic decision-making. The COVID-19 pandemic has amplified these preexisting forms of discrimination.

Methodology

Interviews were conducted in Lagos State from March to June 2021. Lagos State is the most populous state in the southwestern geopolitical zone of Nigeria, with an estimated population of over 24 million people (Lagos State Government n.d.). It remains the economic capital and the financial hub of the nation and is home to the busiest international airport in the country. In addition, Lagos was one of the first states in Nigeria to implement lockdowns and social distancing, with a substantial impact on the economy and livelihoods. Lagos has high levels of urban poverty, with more than two-thirds of the state's population living in informal housing, and more than 380 slum communities spread throughout the state. The COVID-19 pandemic has had a devastating impact on people's livelihoods and access to food in urban slum communities, as a five-week lockdown, an economic downturn, and rising food prices left many households struggling to feed their families.

To provide illustrative examples of how different groups in Lagos were affected, with a specific focus on gender, we interviewed twenty-eight women—twelve residing in urban slum communities, eight informal market traders, and eight women living with disabilities. Participants were recruited through local civil society organizations and snowball sampling. All the interviews were carried out in the respondents' preferred language and in a private and safe location to allow for minimum interruptions during the interviews. Semistructured interviews were conducted around the themes set out by the Gender and COVID-19 Matrix, as described in the introduction to this volume (Gender and COVID-19 Project n.d.). Interviews lasted one hour on average and were audio-recorded and then transcribed. They were independently coded and analyzed using thematic content analysis.

Effects on Paid Work and Financial Security

The imposed lockdowns had a significant impact on women's livelihoods. Many of those engaged in informal market trading experienced business interruptions or losses.

> It affected my business because during the lockdown period, I didn't have anything at home to keep the business running, and there was no way to go to the market and stock up. Since that time, even as the lockdown was relaxed, the cost of everything went up in the market. To get money to buy goods to sell was difficult for me. I just buy in little quantity now. (Monica, widow, forty years old, food stuff seller)

Women traders either could not access supplies to sell or could not afford the increased prices of wholesale goods. As small entrepreneurs without formal networks, they did not have the resources to weather these interruptions. Consequently, one woman trader noted that she was unable to afford the rent at her shop and had to give it up. Another, a single mother living in the slums, struggled to pay rent at home. She explained,

> Basically, there was a time when my house rent expired during the lockdown. I really do not blame the lady; she too needs money. I was actually [pressured] to make provision for the household even with she knows everywhere is on standstill. (Adaeze, unpartnered mother, twenty-seven years old, Makoko community)

There were no programs providing rent relief for homes or businesses to mitigate this insecurity. In April 2020, through the Central Bank of Nigeria, the government introduced a targeted credit facility stimulus package to support households and micro, small, and medium enterprises affected by the COVID-19 pandemic. However, none of the participants in this study benefited from the initiative, as the distribution framework was not designed to reach those most in need.

Women traders were put in the position of having to choose between economic and personal security. To get to informal markets, they often had to cross checkpoints where police monitored curfew and travel restrictions. One woman explained,

> It was never easy to get to the market cos crossing those police checkpoints and all that it was not an easy thing once you don't have that clearance it wasn't an easy stuff because I remembered I was arrested like three times without clearance. (Anulika, partnered, thirty-six years old, provisions seller)

Such arrests could incur financial costs, as money often had to be paid before one was released. Arrests could also put women at risk of police violence, including sexual violence. People with disabilities were particularly affected by business closures, as they had fewer options for generating income. A woman with a disability who had previously volunteered with civil society organizations explained,

> It has affected me because sometimes I could be invited as a facilitator or something programs on family and that will give me little money for my pocket after my transport for me and my taxi, all of those shut down during the pandemic. (Susan, physically challenged, unpartnered, forty years old, disability advocate)

Another woman noted,

> I had a shop before, but now, I am baking from home. No shop again. You know, during the lockdown, the rent was due, and I couldn't pay. All the money I was using for the business, we spent it. So, I am just picking up. (Bukola, visually impaired, widow, forty-seven years old, baker)

While women sought new opportunities to cope with the effects of the lockdown, these too were constrained by the broader economic downturn caused by the pandemic. One woman explained how she tried to diversify into house cleaning but still could not meet her family's financial needs:

> There is pressure for money, I have nothing. I have to leave my shop when there was no money to pay. So, I am working now as a home service and many people too don't have money to call for home service, so I am now on my own. (Oluwatoyin, partnered, forty-five years old, Ilaje community)

Government and nongovernmental organizations attempted to cushion the effect of the COVID-19 lockdown by providing palliatives. Some respondents reported that they received food and household goods donated by religious and nongovernmental organizations. A woman living in a slum noted,

> Yes. The local government chairman brought us rice and beans to share in the community. Aside from that my street chairman also shared rice and egg. A landlord on the street also shared Indomie [instant noodles] for children. (Rekia, unpartnered, forty-five years old, Agege community)

Some respondents commended the government's efforts. A woman living in a slum community noted,

> Government is even trying. Dem try. They even share food in some area, ehn if no be say government say we should sit down for house, this thing wey we dey talk a lot of people for don die. (Raimot, widow, thirty-nine years old, Mushin community)

However, respondents also felt that while the government provision of foodstuffs, cash transfers, and other palliatives was commendable, they could have done better monitoring the distribution process to ensure that the most vulnerable were prioritized. While the policy documents outlining the distribution of palliatives recommended that they should be distributed to "vulnerable" and "poor" households, how this was to be determined was not detailed. Many respondents in need said they did not notice the impact of the government relief efforts. For example, one woman living with a disability commented, "I don't even know what they are doing, so I cannot tell you if they are doing a good job or not. I don't see them doing anything" (Ruth, albino, partnered, forty years old, teacher).

Others compared the Nigerian response to what they heard about other countries in the media. A woman trader said,

> They're not doing enough because, in other countries, we used to hear how they are helping their people, providing food for them, even paying those workers that are not going to work, to help them and make them feel comfortable. (Esther, partnered, thirty-eight years old, baby care product seller)

Many suggested that direct financial relief would have been welcome and would have demonstrated that the government valued their work.

> They should give us a soft loan. You know when we have a soft loan that you have to pay a very soft interest, you'll be encouraged to do more. Giving us grants to support our business because we the women do a lot of support, especially at home. We have to support our husbands because being visually impaired doesn't mean my daughter or son would need something and I won't be able to provide. (Bukola, visually impaired, unpartnered, forty years old, caterer)

Women petty traders also noted that loans with no or low interest would have enabled their businesses to weather the crisis. Without such support, financial insecurity contributed to heightened anxiety and stress. A women trader described the increased mental load:

> The way the economy is now it bothers everybody, it bothers because you check now you see many things now is on the high side, so it makes me, I will use myself, it makes me to put more effort in everything I'm doing just to meet up. (Esther, partnered, thirty-eight years old, baby care product seller)

A woman living with a disability explained how staying at home with no options to earn income caused persistent anxiety, noting,

> Such [issues] arise especially for the fact that I'm not working yet and I have to depend on some friends for help and all so it's not been very easy so to speak. (Mariam, visually impaired, unpartnered mother, thirty years old, lawyer)

Unpaid Care Work

Women reported an increase in household workload during the lockdown, which reduced the time they had to spend on economic activities.

> There was an increase [in household responsibilities]. The children were at home, I use to wash clothes all the time, and then drive them here and there. But if they went to school, they will just go [themselves], and I myself will go to my business. Now they are home and I can't do business. (Jennifer, partnered thirty-five years old, food item seller)

Respondents noted that the workload at home increased due to the need to improve hygiene as a protective measure. A woman with a disability explained that her perceived increased risk of adverse COVID outcomes meant she spent more time ensuring cleanliness:

> I had to be extra neat because of the pandemic. You know, the way you prepare your food and everything. Then the washing of my hands was like times 10 compared to when the pandemic had not come. (Tobiloba, unpartnered, woman with a disability, thirty-five years old, lawyer and disability advocate)

Other women with disabilities experienced reduced care support from others due to distancing policies, increasing the time and effort they had to spend on self-care. However, others found that the increased presence of women family members staying at home allowed a sharing of unpaid care work. A young woman explained, "In (my household), workload actually did not increase because my parents were around and I have understanding and supportive parents, so everybody just shares it amongst themselves" (Alice, eighteen years old, Ikobayo community).

Similarly, mothers explained that their daughters, who were at home because schools were closed, helped with household chores. There was no mention of sons or young men helping with household work, and there were no government or civil society initiatives mentioned that helped ease the burden of unpaid care work.

Still, increased unpaid care heightened anxiety. A single mother explained, "I feel pressured a lot as I am the only one looking after the children. It causes a lot of pressure" (Monica, widow, forty years old, food stuff seller).

Informal market traders expressed stress related to managing increased unpaid care work at the same time that they were trying to overcome business obstacles related to market interruptions. Women with disabilities experienced isolation and loneliness.

> The social distancing, you know, as a person with a disability, you'll need help, you cannot maintain social distance. It has really affected us. It was difficult because people too do not want to help at times. They'll be reluctant. And even myself too, that is why I did not go out for . . . like two months, I stayed at home. (Bukola, visually impaired, widow, forty-seven years old, baker)

Respondents had developed coping mechanisms in response to such stressors. A young woman with a disability explained,

> I know a bit about mental health, so I give myself time to relax, and when they're choking me up I'll just lock myself in my room and watch YouTube videos or just do something to make me feel relaxed. So, I didn't really allow the pressure to hit me. (Oluwamayowa, visually impaired, unpartnered, twenty-one years old, student)

Support for stress among respondents came primarily from family. Women called on family and friends for both emotional support and help with increased care burdens when in need.

Sexual and Gender-Based Violence

Participants were aware that SGBV increased during the lockdown, noting that women, girls, and people with disabilities were most at risk. They felt that the lockdown made it almost impossible for survivors of SGBV to report cases and seek help.

> So, I've spoken to someone who was saying her husband has been beating her, how will she talk about it? No way, nobody understands her. Apart from on a normal basis, persons with a disability goes through a lot of sexual abuse, a lot. So, during that pandemic, it just made them stuck in a position, so they can't even

> run. Where are you running to? You cannot even leave your house. (Adebimpe, visually impaired, unpartnered, thirty years old, entrepreneur)

The identified enablers of SGBV were lack of finances, school closures, poor disability inclusion in programming for SGBV, gender discriminatory norms that make reporting difficult due to the perpetrator's control of victims' access to help, poor security especially in slum communities, stigmatization of survivors, and a lack of adequate penalties for offenders. Respondents noted that while incidents of SGBV had increased, acceptance of such abuse was rooted in persistent cultural norms. A young woman living in a slum explained,

> My neighbor, a girl of 15 years, is being abused by her uncle, but she can't say anything about it because they will not want to bring shame to their family, as Nigerians will put it. (Augusta, nineteen years old, Ilaje community)

Societal norms blaming women for SGBV persisted. One woman expressed,

> In terms of sexual harassment, some of the females dress rough, they do not dress well. You know, once you are not dressing well, you are showing your body to men, and it attracts men. (Favour, partnered, thirty-four years old, food stuff seller)

Lack of justice also enabled ongoing and increased violence:

> Basically, we do not have major ways to protect or help women but if there is a logical or more defined punishment for the assault like for people they catch assaulting a child or a female or a lady but for the fact that there is no defined punishment for it . . . it is about having a very concrete punishment for anybody involved in assault. . . . So it is just the fact that we do not have a very good legal system basically. That is why I feel we are still having this issue. (Adaeze, unpartnered mother, twenty-seven years old, Makoko community)

Persistent cultural norms and a lack of legal redress, combined with the effects of lockdown, increased SGBV, something all respondents were aware of but for which they had few options in terms of response.

Discussion

The COVID-19 pandemic had widespread social and economic effects across Nigeria, which were not experienced equally. The pandemic response caused significant hardships for some of the most marginalized Nigerian women, including those living in slums, working in the informal sector, and living with disabilities. They experienced significant income losses, increased unpaid work, and increased gender-based violence. While the experiences of these effects were nuanced depending on a woman's lived experience across her identity, women faced the same economic marginalization as they experienced the impacts of quasi-universal structural inequalities determined by neoliberal systems of production and validation that prioritize certain groups (i.e., those that contribute most of capital development and production) over others. Given the norms of social and gendered reproduction, this has meant more women than men entered the pandemic in poverty and without the resources or networks to weather a crisis. Concurrently, gender norms dictated that women take on increased care work and fostered conditions for SGBV.

Most respondents reported that their primary concerns during the pandemic were financial. During the pandemic, many faced anxiety and fear about the security of their livelihoods; several women in this study reported reduced income and increased unpaid work, both of which reinforced existing social inequities. This disproportionate impact on women was felt particularly by informal market traders and women living in slum communities. Other studies have reported similar trends (Tan et al. 2021; Ekoh et al. 2020; Ogando, Rogan, and Moussié 2022; Kulkarni et al. 2021). The widespread effects of the pandemic on these women's ability to earn incomes further exaggerated the gender gap and put women and households at increased risk of food insecurity and poverty.

Gendered roles, alongside race, class, sexuality, and patriarchal/capitalist structures, also contribute to creating structural barriers to women joining the formal sector, resulting in women seeking paid work through the informal sector. The informal sector was disproportionately impacted by the pandemic, resulting in women—who make up most workers in the sector's front-facing occupations, such as market traders, hairdressers, and domestic workers—facing significant financial losses. Few participants had alternative sources of income. People living with disabilities faced greater challenges seeking paid work because of the unequal impact on their mobility.

With the lockdowns and the closure of schools, day-care centers, religious organizations, and many formal businesses, women had to balance the sudden increase in unpaid care responsibilities with the need to earn enough money to feed themselves and their families. Several women reported an increased household workload during the pandemic, though some reported that family support and shared responsibilities among female family members may have reduced this impact.

Since the onset of the COVID-19 pandemic, there have been reported increases in cases of gender-based violence. This has been validated by credible organizations, including the Lagos State government-run Domestic and Gender Violence Response Team, which has stated that it received increased reports of sexual and domestic violence after the lockdown started in March 2021. The experiences shared here corroborate these reports, as women in all the subgroups we interviewed reported cases of SGBV. Several risks known to be associated with increased SGBV—such as economic strain, school closures, and reduced access to health and social services—were aggravated by the pandemic.

Such effects on Nigerian women during the crisis were not inevitable. They were structured by preexisting intersectoral and postcolonial inequities and by the persistent bias in policy responses that failed to acknowledge these inequities. As such, they can be rectified by a gender-informed transformative pandemic response and recovery.

One important priority is for social and policy change to prompt more equal distribution of both income-generation opportunities and unpaid care work at the household level between women and men and to prioritize the needs of people with disabilities and other marginalized groups. A shift in perception around gender roles and social norms that disproportionately entrench the burden of child and family care on women and improved childcare options for families with young children could reduce barriers to income-generating activities and improve women's mental health. In cases of economic downturns, such as that caused by policy responses to the pandemic, economic relief intervention should target those most impacted, such as workers in the informal economy and people with disabilities. Gender-balanced financial aid for women, such as non-interest-bearing soft loans for small businesses, could also provide opportunities for empowerment. Similarly, barriers to women entering the formal sector of the labor market would improve resilience in the context of crisis.

Additionally, economic and care support, such as pandemic palliatives from the government and nongovernmental organizations, should be provided equitably, giving priority to informal market traders, those living in slums, and women with disabilities whose mobility can be greatly impacted by pandemic public health regulations. Strategies to proactively prevent and manage SGBV during a pandemic crisis are essential. Examples of these include creating community programs to address social norms against SGBV, strengthening and implementing law enforcement against SGBV, and increasing the number of shelters and helplines for women experiencing SGBV. To reduce the mental health impact of pandemics, increased awareness of positive coping strategies is needed for both men and women. Such programs must be tailored to meet the needs of those most at risk and be buttressed by systemic change to address those factors that put Nigerian women disproportionately at risk during the pandemic.

References

Abayomi, Akinola, Oluwakemi Odukoya, Olamid Okulaja, Olufisayo Okusanya, Adesoji Ologun, Kafayat Ajuwon, Abiola Phillips, et al. 2024. "The Lagos State COVID-19 Think-Tank, a Potential Framework for Decision-Making in a Pandemic Era." *Annals of African Medicine* 23(3):262–266. https://doi.org/10.4103/aam.aam_110_21.

Chimhowu, Admos, Sushila Zeitlyn, and Omowumi Asubiaro Dada. 2012. "Gender in Nigeria Report 2012: Improving the Lives of Girls and Women in Nigeria: Issues, Policies, Action." British Council Nigeria. https://www.researchgate.net/publication/260134459_Gender_in_Nigeria_Report_2012_Improving_the_Lives_of_Girls_and_Women_in_Nigeria_Issues_Policies_Action.

CLGF (Commonwealth Local Government Forum). 2019. "Country Profile 2019: The Local Government System in Nigeria." http://www.clgf.org.uk/default/assets/File/Country_profiles/Nigeria.pdf.

Dan-Nwafor, Chioma, Chinwe Lucia Ochu, Kelly Elimian, John Oladejo, Elsie Ilori, Chukwuma Umeokonkwo, Laura Steinhardt et al. 2020. "Nigeria's Public Health Response to the COVID-19 Pandemic: January to May 2020." *Journal of Global Health* 10 (2): 020399. https://doi.org/10.7189/JOGH.10.020399.

Ekoh, Prince C., Patricia U. Agbawodikeizu, Chukwuemeka Ejimkararonye, Elizabeth O. George, Chigozie D. Ezulike, and Ikechukwu Nnebe. 2020. "COVID-19 in Rural Nigeria: Diminishing Social Support for Older People in Nigeria." *Gerontology and Geriatric Medicine* 6: 1–7. https://doi.org/10.1177%2F2333721420986301.

FAO (Food and Agriculture Organisation of the United Nations). n.d. "Gender and Land Rights Database." https://www.fao.org/land-water/land/land-governance/land-resources-planning-toolbox/category/details/fr/c/1047633/. Accessed March 13, 2025.

Federal Government of Nigeria. 2020. Presidential Task Force on COVID-19: Mid-term Report. https://statehouse.gov.ng/covid19/wp-content/uploads/2020/10/PTF-MTR-SEPT-29.1.pdf.

Gender and COVID-19 Project. n.d. "Gender Matrix: Nigeria." https://www.genderandcovid-19.org/matrix/.

IPU Parline. n.d. "Global Data on National Parliaments: Nigeria." https://data.ipu.org/node/125/elections?chamber_id=13562&election_id=27999.

Kulkarni, Seema, Sneha Bhat, Pallavi Harshe, and Swati Satpute. 2021. "Locked Out of Livelihoods: Impact of COVID-19 on Single Women Farmers in Maharashtra, India." *Economia Politica* 39 (1): 185–202.

Lagos State Government. n.d. "About Lagos." https://lagosstate.gov.ng/.

NPC (National Population Commission) (Nigeria) and ICF. 2019. *Nigeria: 2018 Demographic and Health Survey Key Findings*. Abuja, Nigeria and Rockville, MD: NPC and ICF. https://dhsprogram.com/pubs/pdf/SR264/SR264.pdf.

Ogando, Ana Carolina, Michael Rogan, and Rachel Moussié. 2022. "Impacts of the COVID-19 Pandemic and Unpaid Care Work on Informal Workers' Livelihoods." *International Labour Review* 161 (2): 171–194. https://doi.org/10.1111/ilr.12332.

President, Federal Republic of Nigeria. 2021. "Coronavirus Disease (COVID-19) Health Protection Regulations 2021." https://mlpng.com/covid-19-health-protection-regulations-2021/.

Tan, Heang-Lee, Amy Oyekunle, Uche Ralph-Opara, Erica Rosser, Rosemary Morgan, and Kate Hawkins. 2021. "How Has Nigeria Responded to the Gendered Impacts of COVID-19?" Gender and COVID-19 Project. https://www.genderandcovid-19.org/wp-content/uploads/2021/09/PAC00467_Gender-and-Covid-19-Nigerias-Pandemic-Response.pdf.

UNDP (United Nations Development Program). 2020. "The COVID-19 Pandemic in Nigeria: Potential Impact of Lockdown Policies on Poverty and Well-being—Brief 3." UNDP Nigeria. April 21. https://www.undp.org/nigeria/publications/covid-19-pandemic-nigeria-potential-impact-lockdown-policies-poverty-and-well-being-brief-3.

UNICEF Nigeria. n.d. "Education." https://www.unicef.org/nigeria/education.

United Nations Nigeria. 2020. "Gender-Based Violence in Nigeria during the COVID-19 Crisis: The Shadow Pandemic (Brief, 4 May 2020)." UN Women. https://nigeria.un.org/sites/default/files/2020-05/Gender%20Based%20Violence%20in%20Nigeria%20During%20COVID%2019%20Crisis_The%20Shadow%20Pandemic.pdf.

World Bank. 2022. "Deep Structural Reforms Guided by Evidence Are Urgently Needed to Lift Millions of Nigerians Out of Poverty, Says New World Bank Report." Press release, March 22, 2022. https://www.worldbank.org/en/news/press-release/2022/03/21/afw-deep-structural-reforms-guided-by-evidence-are-urgently-needed-to-lift-millions-of-nigerians-out-of-poverty.

World Economic Forum. 2021. *Global Gender Gap Report 2021: Insight Report*. Switzerland: World Economic Forum. https://www3.weforum.org/docs/WEF_GGGR_2021.pdf.

9 "I Feel Like I've Been Left at 'Good Luck. Hopefully, Nothing Goes Wrong'": The Experiences of Pregnant Women during COVID-19 in the UK

Asha Herten Crabb, Karen Grépin, and Clare Wenham

Introduction

During the first year of the pandemic, the UK reported 3.91 million COVID-19 cases, 401,425 hospitalizations and 76,723 deaths. Although the peak of the worst wave of COVID-19 occurred in January 2021, the first year of the pandemic was arguably more chaotic, as the government and the population came to grips with the threat at hand, developed new ways of living and working at home, and followed guidance from the government to limit social contacts through school and workplace closures and two nationwide lockdowns. In addition to the health effects of the pandemic, the economic and social effects of these nonpharmaceutical interventions were substantial. To mitigate some of these externalities, the government introduced a furlough scheme for those unable to work and increased universal credit payments for those in receipt of them. In addition, the three devolved administrations and the central government of the UK developed and published thousands of policy documents to reflect new ways of living and to support individuals and communities through the pandemic mire.

Despite these interventions to protect people from health, social, and economic vulnerabilities, women, and notably pregnant women, remained notably absent in government planning and consideration. This in turn reflects the dominant patriarchal structures of governance that were reproduced globally in governments' responses to the COVID-19 pandemic, whereby a prioritization of national security logic sought to protect the state and its economy against the threat of a health emergency, which in turn meant that social and governmental provisions relied on essentialist understandings of life and death. Consequently, governments rationed health resources and grappled with the sometimes-conflicting priorities of economic stability versus public health. Such policies UK's failed to consider the myriad ways in which structural inequalities pervade society and limit women's public and private participation. These were further challenging for those with a range of intersecting identities that are hampered by structural factors. Many of these policies had particular effects on pregnant women. Disruption or changes to the provision of maternal health services can have devastating effects on maternal and neonatal health outcomes. During the Ebola outbreak in West Africa, reduced utilization of maternity health services in Sierra Leone translated to an estimated 3,600 additional maternal deaths, a number comparable to direct Ebola mortality (Sochas, Channon, and Nam 2017). During the outbreak in Eastern Democratic Republic of the Congo, women avoided accessing assisted delivery, fearing that any bleeding would be conflated with Ebola and thus they would be isolated from family and potentially exposed to the virus (McKay et al. 2020). During the Zika epidemic in Brazil, although utilization of maternal health services increased, given the clinical presentation of the virus's sequelae in neonates, worse health outcomes were observed, including increased rates of premature birth, miscarriage, and further obstetric complications (Brasil et al. 2016). This type of situation is mirrored in high-income settings: during SARS in 2003, women in Hong Kong altered their birth plans to facilitate their partners' participation.

Disruption to maternity care during COVID-19 was no exception. Every country and clinic had to make difficult decisions about which health services to continue and which to alter, reduce, or cancel in order to reallocate clinical, human, and financial resources to COVID-19, as well as to reduce the risk of disease transmission within clinical settings (WHO 2020b; Roberton et al. 2020). In the absence of UK government policy in the early stages of the pandemic, the Royal College of Obstetricians and Gynaecologists (RCOG), a membership body that regulates and licenses obstetricians and gynecologists, issued guidelines suggesting that it was essential to maintain antenatal, intrapartum, and postpartum care for all pregnant women, including those with suspected or confirmed cases of COVID-19 (RCOG 2020a). However, one-third of maternal units in the UK implemented policies to reduce inpatient stays during the postpartum period to reduce the burden on services and decrease the risk of disease transmission (Rimmer, Al Wattar, and Members 2020). In the absence of a clear government position, decisions were decentralized to the level of each NHS trust (the unit of geographic and governance decentralization within the UK's National Health Service), which led to wide variation in how care was provided during the first year of the pandemic. Pregnant women reported having appointments cancelled (Lebel et al. 2020) or transitioned away from clinics to telephone or virtual consultations (Rimmer et al. 2020), which in turn affected the comprehensiveness of information they disclosed to the clinician (Karavadra et al. 2020). Women also noted reduced midwife and health visitor access in the community (Karavadra et al. 2020), the suspension of labor induction and elective caesarean sections, and the revision of birth plans with zoned COVID-19 and non-COVID-19 wards. In addition, in many NHS trusts, birth partners were not permitted during antepartum care or until the last stages of the delivery process, if at all, which was perceived to have exacerbated pregnant women's mental burden, anxiety, and stress (Lebel et al. 2020; Karavadra et al. 2020).

While the International Federation of Gynaecology and Obstetrics recommended that birthing partners not be permitted to attend births, in order to reduce risk exposure (Poon et al. 2020), the RCOG championed partners being permitted throughout pregnancy and labor interactions, noting the benefits it brings to the woman in labor and to the resulting health outcomes (RCOG 2020b). However, due to lockdown and self-isolation policies related to COVID-19, many partners faced additional challenges in accessing maternity services as support to pregnant women. Thus, there was a discrepancy between the continuity of care that RCOG recommended and the reality on the ground in maternity services across the country in the absence of clear policy from the Department of Health and Social Care and NHS England, which in turn led to large divergences between trusts in service provision.

This gap between policy and reality risked wide-reaching effects on maternal health outcomes: attendance at antenatal care is directly linked to positive outcomes (Dowswell et al. 2015), and 70 percent of maternity clinics reported a reduction in antenatal appointments in 2020 (Jardine et al. 2021). Early data highlighted an increase in stillbirths in the UK during the first wave of the pandemic, although without a causal link to reduced service utilization, but disruption to health services likely played some role (Khalil et al. 2020). Italian research painted a similar picture, with a threefold increase in stillbirths (De Curtis, Villani, and Polo 2020). Yet a subsequent analysis of UK stillbirth numbers from April to June 2020 revealed no significant difference compared to 2019 (Stowe et al. 2021). While research on the effects of service modifications on physical health conditions is currently inconclusive, there was a surge in distress and psychological conditions among pregnant women during COVID-19 compared to prepandemic cohorts (Lebel et al. 2020; Cameron et al. 2020). Moreover, given that prior to the pandemic there was increasing evidence of the discrepancy in maternal outcomes between white, Black, and minority ethnic women, with Black women up to four times more likely to die in UK maternity provision than their white counterparts (Knight 2022), we can only imagine that such negative externalities were amplified by the pandemic.

Given this context and the gap between RCOG guidance and the reality within NHS trusts, we sought to understand the impact of COVID-19 on pregnant women's perceptions of their childbirth experiences in the UK. Using qualitative data from sequential interviews conducted over six months, we analyzed the key impacts of policy changes during COVID-19 on how women interacted with maternal health services and how this, in turn, affected their experience of pregnancy during the pandemic.

Methods

As per the methodology in the introduction to this book, semistructured phone interviews were conducted with twenty-three women who identified as pregnant or as new mothers in April and May 2020. The same participants were recontacted and invited for a second interview in October and November 2020. From our initial sample, fourteen agreed to a follow-up interview.

Those interviewed self-identified as women between twenty-five and fifty years old and, although this was not an inclusion criterion, all were in heterosexual relationships. We did not purposefully recruit women from different ethnic, socioeconomic, geographical, and political backgrounds, which was, in hindsight, a design flaw. Noting, however, the challenges of doing so with the recruitment methods in the early months of the pandemic, online via social media adverts, women self-selected to participate. Where we have data on their ethnicity or geography, or other demographic factors discussed in the course of the interview, we recorded this. Cognizant of the time required to participate in an interview, we envision that most women were from higher socioeconomic groups and not in the frontline workforce. Once the interview recordings were transcribed, we undertook a framework analysis of the data collected (Ritchie et al. 2013). Two researchers reviewed a subsample of the transcripts, identified key themes in the data, created a unified codebook, and applied it to the remaining dataset. New themes identified during the application process were added iteratively to the codebook. Once compiled, the framework was subjected to second-order analysis to narrow down the scope of themes to those related to pregnancy, maternity care, and ante- and postnatal support. The second-order analysis was undertaken to find synergies across the two datasets and identify key messages.

Results and Findings

The women interviewed expressed concern about the impact of the pandemic on their pregnancies. We classified their concerns into three categories: concerns about quality healthcare provision, the absence of birth partners, and limitations on broader support adding to their anxiety.

Concerns about Quality Healthcare Provision

Despite RCOG guidance, almost all the women interviewed stated that routine antenatal services had changed because of the pandemic. This ranged depending on NHS trust but included examples such as the following:

> They gave me a blood pressure kit to do at home. (woman, forty, mixed race, London)

> I was meant to go for cervical length ultrasound at 16 weeks and they said because of the outbreak we're going to roll that in with your 21-week scan. (woman, thirty-five, white-British, Scotland)

> I haven't had any blood taken for 12 weeks. (woman, thirty-four, white-British, Bristol)

One woman, who was overweight and, as a consequence, was told she would get additional care during pregnancy, said, "To be honest, I haven't seen a damn midwife since this has started" (woman, age thirty-seven, white-British, London).

Another, who had been through assisted reproductive processes, stated,

> I was meant to go in for a blood test so that I could wean myself off injectable progesterone that I was taking every day, and that got shut down. So . . . they said, "you're just going to have to keep going for another four weeks of injections because we can't ask to see if your levels are high enough." (woman, thirty-five, white-British, Scotland)

This lack of direct interaction with antenatal services meant the potential for missed concerns. One woman described in detail the missed appointments leading her to feel unsupported during her pregnancy: "Because of the pandemic, the 16-week appointment was a telephone appointment. . . . And then the 25-week appointment and the 28-week appointment [were] rolled in together" (woman, thirty-two, white-British, Lincoln).

This left some to seek care through informal channels with friends who had some health-related knowledge. As one respondent who herself had healthcare knowledge narrated,

> I get a lot of fairly frantic WhatsApp messages, which I have no problem with. And I'll answer if I can, like one of the women ended up, got a positive COVID test. . . . [she asked] "Am I still able to go to the birth center?" because . . . she tried to call her midwife but you know, they're only working Monday to Friday and she was just really scared. (woman, thirty-seven, white-British, Scotland)

This feeling of being unsupported continued in the postpartum period, with women concerned about their interaction with community-based services and GPs:

> I had to go to the GP for a blood pressure check-up . . . I was waiting outside. The GP was running 40 minutes late and I was still only three weeks post-surgery. So, I popped to the desk and said, "Is there any chance I could pop in and sit down? Because I'm finding it difficult standing outside." and she said "Well, you can come in, but you can't sit down." . . . And I was in there [with the doctor] for all of three minutes. And she said "How are you?" And I said, "Well, I'm a bit you know, quite upset. . . . I don't think it's reasonable to make people who have had surgery or babies wait outside in the cold. There's not a lot of humanity been applied." (woman, thirty-four, white-other, southwest England)

Others suffered from gaps in community care appointments, leading women to improvise: "I had to resort to weighing him by putting him in an Ikea bag, and using luggage scales" (woman, forty-two, white-other, northwest England).

This left many to feel concerned about their pregnancy or postpartum period: "It does make you feel a bit more apprehensive I think, because obviously, you know, you're not getting the same sort of care that you normally get" (woman, thirty-seven, white-British, London).

Another respondent said,

> I feel like I've been left at "good luck. Hopefully, nothing goes wrong. See you when you give birth." And that's been hard. That's possibly been the hardest part of it, being pregnant during all of this, is I've not had those appointments, that I'm a first-time mum, so I have no idea what I'm looking out for. (woman, thirty-seven, white-other, London)

While the situations described above are all changes to supply-side delivery of care, some women also chose to reduce interaction with care providers because of their perception of risk of COVID-19 infection.

> I debated not going, because . . . I'm putting myself at risk going, but then I think it's probably quite unnecessary. (woman, twenty-seven, white-other, Glasgow)

> I didn't really want to go to the hospital or the midwife just because of all the stuff going on. And because I've had a low-risk pregnancy before and this time around, I just kind of like been a bit more blasé about it. (woman, twenty-nine, white-British, Leicestershire)

This was amplified by inconsistent policies between NHS trusts, so that women did not know why their care providers might allow something that others might not; changes to trust policy were commonplace throughout 2020. Many women changed plans for birth as a result of supply disruption and demand changes and on account of changing provisions within trusts:

> When the pandemic happened, we kind of thought, let's go for the C-section, because it gives us a bit more control of timing. (woman, forty-eight, white-British, Suffolk)

> On the 20th of March, they closed the home birth team [and said] "the ambulance service can't support us and also our staffing, we need to make sure that people are safe and in hospitals first and foremost." (woman, thirty-five, white-British, Reading)

This variability also transpired in postpartum care, whereby different boroughs had differing policies on in-person care.

> GPs in Lambeth [a borough of London], they're all open, he just assumed that I've been having weekly checks or, . . . But because I'm in Wandsworth [another borough of London], nothing has opened up. (woman, thirty-three, white-British, London)

Absence of Birth Partners

Most women described distress about rules restricting the attendance of birth partners throughout their maternity interactions, despite this not being recommended by RCOG. While this policy varied over time and by NHS trust, it had negative impacts on most women's experiences of their healthcare provision.

Some women lamented that partners could not attend scans to provide emotional support and to participate in the process:

> I had to go into the hospital yesterday for some extra monitoring because I was slightly concerned about something. Obviously a very anxious time for both of us—because I don't see this just as my pregnancy—because my husband had to wait in the car park, and I just think that the effect and the impact on him is probably bigger than even on me. (woman, thirty-four, white-other, southwest England).

> I was more sad for him . . . he just said, "Well, if we have more kids I'll see the next ones." (woman, thirty-six, white-British, Wales)

Several women expressed their anxieties about being alone while receiving bad news at antenatal scans:

> If there had been anything wrong, I'd have been on my own. And you know that-that-that-that was quite difficult. (woman, thirty-eight, white-other, London)

> As soon as we went to the lobby of the hospital there was a woman there saying no men allowed, you have to stay out, and for me that was really upsetting. . . . I'm sorry. . . . I don't speak about it without crying. I'm going to be emotional—I wasn't sure the baby was still alive. (woman, twenty-four, white-British, London)

This limitation on partners' attendance made some decide to seek private care, which they might otherwise not have:

> What we've also done is we booked a private scan. We've done it in a place where they allowed partners, so we do that on purpose for him to be able to see the baby. (woman, twenty-four, white-British, London)

One woman was met with resistance when she asked a consultant (MD) if she could call her husband so they could discuss delivery options together after finding out her baby was breach:

> I had to have a conversation about [some complications] and had to do all of that consultation on my own . . . I did actually put my foot down with a consultant and say please can I call my husband so we can go through this together. (woman, thirty-four, white-other, southwest England).

Several women extrapolated this concern to the role that partners play as advocates during pregnancy:

> I am . . . very concerned about my ability to advocate for my own care. I know that, as it stands, if things are very straightforward my husband will be able to be there for the majority of that period of time, but there will definitely be a time after the baby's born when he can't be present. And I am concerned that I'd really be relying on him to know what I want to be done. (woman, thirty, white-British, Berkshire)

> I'm quite nervous about the concept of basically having to go through a large part of labor potentially on my own or if something goes wrong, not having someone

there to advocate for me if I'm in a huge amount of pain. (woman, forty-two, white-other, northwest England)

These women expressed distress about the postpartum experience, where they were left alone overnight with limited help with the baby or with their own care. Several women told us they had left the hospital within twenty-four hours not on medical advice, but to leave an unbearable situation:

So Tuesday morning at 2 A.M. we had, I had, an emergency C-section. And then because the preeclampsia really kicked in, I was there for another week and a day without him so this is I guess this is where kind of the COVID stuff really hits home. Um, so my husband was allowed to be there for, you know, the surgery and he was able to be with [the baby] and I. For me it was like four or five hours or something after the birth, I'm a little hazy on details, um, but then he had to leave. . . . I was on so much medication. I was so exhausted, and then I couldn't, I didn't have [my husband] there. . . . So there was this dread. (woman, forty, mixed race, London)

Support Outside the Health Sector

Women had imagined that they would be able to prepare for becoming a parent as part of the ritual of pregnancy and new motherhood, which they were no longer able to enjoy:

I think about missing the fun things that are supposed to happen when you're pregnant. Like a baby shower, and going shopping for a stroller, and stuff like that. Such minor issues compared to what most people are dealing with, but it's just—you look forward to these things. (woman, forty-five, white-other, Scotland)

Others feared that they wouldn't be able to introduce their new baby to the family:

I have worried about [the] extended family . . . wanting to come and see the new baby and just the kind of politics of handling that and how I feel about that and the kind of risks associated with that. (woman, twenty-seven, white-other, Glasgow)

Women expressed that this might not only affect the family, but that it would cause them anxiety and deprive them of help readjusting in the postpartum period.

This concern also echoed in regard to some women's lack of ability to establish a social support group for a new phase in life:

How I'm going to handle being on my own with a new baby without that kind of—without the connections that I would normally have expected to build up through face-to-face antenatal classes . . . I'm concerned about how isolating that could end up being. (woman, forty-two, white-other, northwest England)

One woman with this concern said,

I kind of feel that I've been a bit robbed of the experience . . . we partly live our pregnancies through the eyes of other people around us, and the fact that it's just me and my husband, I mean, a lot of people at work still don't know that I'm pregnant. (woman, thirty-four, white-British, London)

Yet some saw social distancing as a net benefit for their new family dynamics:

I think we've been quite lucky to have this time that we've just dedicated to the baby. You know, we haven't had any other distractions going on since we have been in lockdown.

I've also read that there are some potential positives around breastfeeding, bonding and having that uninterrupted time at home. (woman, thirty-six, white-other, Leicester)

The consolidation of these three factors meant that women had various concerns about having a baby amid a pandemic: "I think it's normal in pregnancy to worry about your baby. . . . But when you've got all day to think about things it definitely becomes more, like, obvious. (woman, twenty-five, British Asian, Leeds)"

Discussion

Pregnancy is a major life event that brings anxiety even under normal circumstances. However, the challenges for women who gave birth in the UK in 2020 were perceived to have been exacerbated by COVID-19 and the absence of formal UK government policy on how to treat them in healthcare settings. This resulted in their healthcare interactions and healthcare utilization being determined by (patriarchal) institutional structures within NHS trusts, which led to a discrepancy between guidance created by RCOG and the reality of the NHS trust response. Our findings highlight women's increased anxieties around access to, and quality of, maternal health services and about birth partners' ability to join them there, as well as women's mixed perceptions regarding the limitations of social support given government lockdown policies. These findings support the growing number of quantitative studies showing that the disruption to maternal health services during COVID-19 resulted in additional anxiety for women during pregnancy (Moyer et al. 2020; Wu et al. 2020; Mortazavi and Ghardashi 2021; Ravaldi et al. 2021; Molgora and Accordini 2020; Vazquez-Vazquez et al. 2021). These findings also contribute greater insight into the broader impacts on women's experiences of pregnancy during the COVID-19 pandemic and the impact of government policy (or lack thereof) on women. We lament the lack of meaningful data to demonstrate the difference of experiences of women of different racial, geographic or other determinant categories of being pregnant or having a newborn during the pandemic in 2020.

As our data reveal, many women felt that they were not getting the quality or quantity of care they desired during COVID-19. The decision by NHS trusts to develop local policy concerning continuity of maternity services left a significant gap in antenatal, intrapartum, and postpartum care. NHS trusts departed from both WHO and RCOG guidance for the pandemic response, which highlights the need to maintain services for pregnant women during pandemics (RCOG 2020b; WHO 2018). The lack of consistency between high-level policies and individual trust responses resulted in women feeling unsupported and overlooked:

> It does feel like pregnant women have been very much overlooked . . . I'm very grateful for the Royal College of Obstetricians and their guidance, because without that, I think we would have been completely adrift . . . it's kind of like, "Good luck, guys. Off you go." (woman, thirty-eight, white-other, London)

This departure from RCOG guidance and the neglect of women are part of a broader narrative of the UK government's failure to understand the gendered nature of pandemics (Herten-Crabb and Wenham 2021). The UK government's consideration of pregnant women during COVID-19 policymaking was limited to classifying them as clinically vulnerable, thus requiring these women to shield and legalizing self-managed medical abortion at home (Parsons and Romanis 2021). Thus, the considerations of these decisions' impacts on pregnant women were not a driver in the decision-making, and this lack of broader policy consideration meant a wholly unsatisfactory experience for women who were pregnant during the pandemic. This was particularly true for Black, Asian, and minority ethnic women in the UK who suffered greater health disparities during pregnancy during the pandemic (Esegbona-Adeigbe 2020), notably that pregnant women from a Black, Asian, or minority ethnic background were more likely to be hospitalized with COVID than their white counterparts (Knight et al. 2020). Our data show that not only was the local provision of maternity services reduced, moved online, or ceased entirely but that many women did not want to interact with maternity services due to concerns about disease transmission. This latter point is consistent with overall levels of other services, such as emergency departments, during COVID-19 (Garrafa et al. 2020), in keeping with previous evidence to this effect from Ebola outbreaks (McKay et al. 2019).

Research conducted through freedom of information requests has elicited information on trusts' policies on birth partner attendance (Coulter and Richards 2020): of eighty-one trusts, seventy-three (90.1 percent) banned partners attending twelve-week scans and seventy-one (87.7 percent) did so for the twenty-week scan. Forty trusts (49.4 percent) banned partners from attending any postnatal service, while eighty (98.8 percent) trusts restricted partners' attendance in some way. Most trusts reported using national guidance and local policies from a range of services in making their decisions, all of which were in some way intended to reduce the risk to healthcare workers by reducing the presence of nonessential attendees at medical appointments. As such, there appears to have been a tension between providing the best care to women utilizing services and protecting NHS staff from potential exposure to COVID-19. Birth partners play an essential role in providing emotional support throughout the perinatal process. Birth partner attendance has been linked to the prevention of postnatal depression, shorter labors, and decreased negative feelings about the experience of childbirth (WHO 2020a). Moreover, structural and systemic racism within maternity provision in NHS trusts has amplified challenges for Black women accessing quality care (Williams, McKail, and Arshad 2023). Our research complements this and contributes to highlighting the inappropriateness of the blanket policy applied by most NHS trusts restricting birth partner attendance at antenatal scans, up until established labor and during the immediate postpartum period in the hospital.

One woman summarized the thoughts of many around the logic of the birth partner rules:

> Not letting the partners in can really lead to some women having, well, mental health issues . . . if you're going for your first scan, or even the second scan, and then you're told either that your pregnancy is not viable, or the fetus is dead in there, or there's a serious deformity or something, and you're by yourself, I just can't imagine having to go through that. And also, I mean, most of the partners

live with the pregnant person. So if they have COVID, the partner has COVID as well. (woman, forty, white-other, southwest England)

Her views are echoed by many (Murphy 2020; Black et al. 2020; Kearns 2020). Indeed, on December 14, 2020, after this research had been undertaken, NHS England updated its policy on birth partners, allowing a support person to be with a pregnant woman throughout all perinatal care (NHS 2020).

There is growing evidence of links between prenatal stress and birth experiences, postnatal depression, and child development. Chronic stress in pregnant women has been linked to increased risk of preterm births (Latendresse 2009). Maternal mental health problems are an independent influencer of infant growth and are associated with ethnicity and deprivation (Traviss, West, and House 2012). Moreover, postnatal depression has been correlated with experiencing traumatic events before and during pregnancy and lack of social support as perceived by the women themselves (Doyle and Klein 2020). This is important when considering the policy implications of restricted health services for pregnant women and new mums and also for their babies: maternal postnatal depression is linked to cognitive and behavioral issues in children (Bernard-Bonnin 2004; Mennes et al. 2009). Research will be required to understand the longer-term implications of women's perceptions of the challenges of pregnancy during a pandemic, particularly in the context of UK policymaking.

In addition to direct impacts on health service provision, UK policies included strict limitations to extra-household gatherings. Only in September 2020 was guidance published allowing single parents and those living alone to create a social support "bubble" with one other household. The ban on gatherings also included an initial ban on support groups, although such mother-baby groups were exempted from regulation for the second national lockdown in November 2020. Our findings highlight the mixed impacts of these policies, with some women suffering from a lack of external, and expected, social support from family and infant support groups while others relished the opportunity to cocoon with their partner and new baby. A perceived lack of social support before and after childbirth is correlated with increased risks to maternal and fetal outcomes as well as postnatal depression and anxiety (Jago, Singh, and Moretti 2020). Higher levels of perceived social support have been found to be a protective factor against anxiety and depression among pregnant women during the COVID-19 pandemic (Lebel et al. 2020).

Conclusion

Our findings reflect the broader gendered structural limitations that we see across the case studies in this book, in that the global political economy and national security policy pathway in epidemic response created a predetermined policy pathway to respond to the pandemic—a pathway focused on protecting the economy and protecting public health at the expense of broader social inequalities, such as those related to gender. Furthermore, our data help to expose and highlight the differences between the public health recommendations from RCOG and WHO and the local-level decision-making by NHS trusts because of governmental policy lacunae. The negative experiences of and impacts on pregnant women during the first year of the COVID-19 pandemic are not inevitable during a public health crisis but, rather, are the consequence of the gendered power hierarchies and structures that dominate the UK government, and particularly the Johnson administration. Local policy affected the delivery of care, often in the absence of evidence as to why interventions were implemented, and have left women with high levels of anxiety and potentially poor maternal health outcomes as a consequence. Many of these will only be realized in due time, given that birth experiences often have long-lasting effects on women. For these reasons, policymakers need to be more cognizant of the reality of women's experiences as policy is created. We recommend that before changes are made to maternity policy, due consultation should be carried out with women experiencing the downstream effects of policy change. While the pandemic is an extraordinary event, and difficult trade-offs need to be made in resource allocation, many of the changes to maternity provision are not costly to implement, such as permitting the presence of birth partners. Yet the costs of not permitting this, in terms of longer-term mental health support for the women affected, may be considerably greater. More fundamentally, this research contributes to the literature from previous outbreaks, including Ebola and Zika, showing that maternity policy should be protected during health emergencies. Policymakers should think creatively about how to continue health services—for example, by using alternative premises and activities to reduce exposure in health settings. By putting women at the center of policymaking during health emergencies, different policy pathways may develop, offering greater sustained support to women so that their maternal safety and experience is not a casualty of prioritizing disease control.

References

Bernard-Bonnin, Anne-Claude. 2004. "Maternal Depression and Child Development." *Paediatrics & Child Health* 9 (8): 575–598. https://doi.org/10.1093/pch/9.8.575.

Black, Benjamin, Jane Laking, and Gillian McKay. 2020. "Birth Partners Are Not a Luxury." *BMJ Opinion* (blog). September 24. https://blogs.bmj.com/bmj/2020/09/24/birth-partners-are-not-a-luxury/.

Brasil, Patrícia, José P. Pereira, Jr., M. Elisabeth Moreira, Rita M. Ribeiro Nogueira, Luana Damasceno, Mayumi Wakimoto, Renata S. Rabello, et al. 2016. "Zika Virus Infection in Pregnant Women in Rio de Janeiro." *New England Journal of Medicine* 375 (24): 2321–2334. https://doi.org/10.1056/NEJMoa1602412.

Cameron, Emily E., Kayla M. Joyce, Chantal P. Delaquis, Kristin Reynolds, Jennifer L. P. Protudjer, and Leslie E. Roos. 2020. "Maternal Psychological Distress & Mental Health Service Use during the COVID-19 Pandemic." *Journal of Affective Disorders* 276: 765–774. https://doi.org/10.1016/j.jad.2020.07.081.

Coulter, Angela, and Tessa Richards. 2020. "Care during COVID-19 Must Be Humane and Person Centred." *BMJ: British Medical Journal* 370: m3483. https://doi.org/10.1136/bmj.m3483.

De Curtis, Mario, Leonardo Villani, and Anna Polo. 2020. "Increase of Stillbirth and Decrease of Late Preterm Infants during the COVID-19 Pandemic Lockdown." *Archives of Disease in Childhood, Fetal and Neonatal Edition* 106 (4): 456. https://doi.org/10.1136/archdischild-2020-320682.

Dowswell, Therese, Guillermo Carroli, Lelia Duley, Simon Gates, A. Metin Gülmezoglu, Dina Khan-Neelofur, and Gilda Piaggio. 2015. "Alternative versus Standard Packages of Antenatal Care for Low-Risk Pregnancy." *Cochrane Database of Systematic Reviews* 7. https://doi.org/10.1002/14651858.CD000934.pub3.

Doyle, Frances Lee, and Louis Klein. 2020. "Postnatal Depression Risk Factors: An Overview of Reviews to Inform COVID-19 Research, Clinical, and Policy Priorities." *Frontiers in Global Women's Health* 22: 577273. https://doi.org/10.3389/fgwh.2020.577273.

Esegbona-Adeigbe, S. 2020. "COVID-19 and the Risk to Black, Asian and Minority Ethnic Women during Pregnancy." *British Journal of Midwifery* 28 (10): 718–723.

Garrafa, Emirena, Rosella Levaggi, Raffaele Miniaci, and Ciro Paolillo. 2020. "When Fear Backfires: Emergency Department Accesses during the COVID-19 Pandemic." *Health Policy* 124 (12): 1333–1339. https://doi.org/10.1016/j.healthpol.2020.10.006.

Herten-Crabb, Asha, and Clare Wenham. 2021. "'I Was Facilitating Everybody Else's Life. And Mine Had Just Ground to a Halt': The COVID-19 Pandemic and its Impact on Women in the United Kingdom." *Social Politics: International Studies in Gender, State & Society* 29 (4): 1213–1235. https://doi.org/10.1093/sp/jxac006.

Jago, Caitlin Anne, Sukhbir Sony Singh, and Felipe Moretti. 2020. "Coronavirus Disease 2019 (COVID-19) and Pregnancy: Combating Isolation to Improve Outcomes." *Obstetrics & Gynecology* 136 (1): 33–36. https://doi.org/10.1097/AOG.0000000000003946.

Jardine, Jennifer, Sophie Relph, Laura A. Magee, Peter von Dadelszen, Edward Morris, Mary Ross-Davie, Tim Draycott, and Asma Khalil. 2021. "Maternity Services in the UK during the Coronavirus Disease 2019 Pandemic: A National Survey of Modifications to Standard Care." *BJOG: An International Journal of Obstetrics & Gynaecology* 128 (5): 880–889. https://doi.org/10.1111/1471-0528.16547.

Karavadra, Babu, Andrea Stockl, Edward Prosser-Snelling, Paul Simpson, and Edward Morris. 2020. "Women's Perceptions of COVID-19 and Their Healthcare Experiences: A Qualitative Thematic Analysis of a National Survey of Pregnant Women in the United Kingdom." *BMC Pregnancy and Childbirth* 20 (1): 600. https://doi.org/10.1186/s12884-020-03283-2.

Kearns, Alicia. 2020. "Alicia Kearns MP Leads Campaign against Lone Births." Press release, September 14. https://www.aliciakearns.com/news/alicia-kearns-mp-leads-campaign-against-lone-births.

Khalil, Asma, Peter von Dadelszen, Tim Draycott, Austin Ugwumadu, Pat O'Brien, and Laura Magee. 2020. "Change in the Incidence of Stillbirth and Preterm Delivery During the COVID-19 Pandemic." *JAMA* 324 (7): 705–706. https://doi.org/10.1001/jama.2020.12746.

Knight, Marian. 2022. "MBRRACE-UK Update: Key Messages from the UK and Ireland Confidential Enquiries into Maternal Death and Morbidity 2021." *Obstetrician & Gynaecologist* 24 (1): 79–81.

Latendresse, Gwen. 2009. "The Interaction Between Chronic Stress and Pregnancy: Preterm Birth from A Biobehavioral Perspective." *Journal of Midwifery & Women's Health* 54 (1): 8–17. https://doi.org/10.1016/j.jmwh.2008.08.001.

Lebel, Catherine, Anna MacKinnon, Mercedes Bagshawe, Lianne Tomfohr-Madsen, and Gerald Giesbrecht. 2020. "Elevated Depression and Anxiety Symptoms among Pregnant Individuals during the COVID-19 Pandemic." *Journal of Affective Disorders* 277: 5–13. https://doi.org/10.1016/j.jad.2020.07.126.

McKay, Gillian, Benjamin Black, and Alice Janvrin. 2019. *Not All that Bleeds Is Ebola: How the DRC Outbreak Impacts Reproductive Health.* New York: International Rescue Committee. https://www.rescue.org/sites/default/files/document/4416/srhebolareport1172020.pdf.

McKay, Gillian, Benjamin Black, Alice Janvrin, and Erin Wheeler. 2020. "Sexual and Reproductive Health in Ebola Response: A Neglected Priority." Humanitarian Practice

Network, March 25. https://odihpn.org/publication/sexual-and-reproductive-health-in-ebola-response-a-neglected-priority/.

Mennes, Maarten, Bea Van den Bergh, Lieven Lagae, and Peter Stiers. 2009. "Developmental Brain Alterations in 17-Year-Old Boys Are Related to Antenatal Maternal Anxiety." *Clinical Neurophysiology* 120 (6): 1116–1122. https://doi.org/10.1016/j.clinph.2009.04.003.

Molgora, Sara, and Monica Accordini. 2020. "Motherhood in the Time of Coronavirus: The Impact of the Pandemic Emergency on Expectant and Postpartum Women's Psychological Well-Being." *Frontiers in Psychology* 11: 567155. https://doi.org/10.3389/fpsyg.2020.567155.

Mortazavi, Forough, and Fatemeh Ghardashi. 2021. "The Lived Experiences of Pregnant Women during COVID-19 Pandemic: A Descriptive Phenomenological Study." *BMC Pregnancy and Childbirth* 21: 193. https://doi.org/10.21203/rs.3.rs-103717/v1.

Moyer, Cheryl A., Sarah D. Compton, Elizabeth Kaselitz, and Maria Muzik. 2020. "Pregnancy-Related Anxiety during COVID-19: A Nationwide Survey of 2740 Pregnant Women." *Archives of Women's Mental Health* 23 (6): 757–765.

Murphy, Gemma. 2020. "RCM and RCOG Urge NHS England to Publish Guidance on Partners during Pregnancy." Royal College of Midwives. Press release, September 8. https://pre.rcm.org.uk/media-releases/2020/september/rcm-and-rcog-urge-nhs-england-to-publish-guidance-on-partners-during-pregnancy/.

Parsons, Jordan A., and Elizabeth C. Romanis. 2021. "2020 Developments in the Provision of Early Medical Abortion by Telemedicine in the UK." *Health Policy* 125 (1): 17–21. https://doi.org/10.1016/j.healthpol.2020.11.006.

Poon, Liona C., Huixia Yang, Anil Kapur, Nir Melamed, Blami Dao, Hema Divakar, H. David McIntyre, et al. 2020. "Global Interim Guidance on Coronavirus Disease 2019 (COVID-19) during Pregnancy and Puerperium from FIGO and Allied Partners: Information for Healthcare Professionals." *International Journal of Gynaecology and Obstetrics* 149 (3): 273–286. https://doi.org/10.1002/ijgo.13156.

Ravaldi, Claudia, Alyce Wilson, Valdo Ricca, Caroline Homer, and Alfredo Vannacci. 2021. "Pregnant Women Voice their Concerns and Birth Expectations during the COVID-19 Pandemic in Italy." *Women and Birth* 34 (4): 335–343. https://doi.org/10.1016/j.wombi.2020.07.002.

RCOG (Royal College of Obstetricians and Gynaecologists). 2020a. "COVID-19 and Pregnancy." *BMJ* 369: m1672. https://doi.org/10.1136/bmj.m1672.

RCOG (Royal College of Obstetricians and Gynaecologists). 2020b. "Coronavirus (COVID-19) Infection in Pregnancy." RCOG. https://www.rcog.org.uk/media/ftzilsfj/2022-12-15-coronavirus-covid-19-infection-in-pregnancy-v16.pdf.

Rimmer, Michael. P., and Bassel H. Al Wattar on behalf of UKARCOG members. 2020. "Provision of Obstetrics and Gynaecology Services during the COVID-19 Pandemic: A Survey of Junior Doctors in the UK National Health Service." *BJOG: An International Journal of Obstetrics & Gynaecology* 127 (9): 1123–1128. https://doi.org/10.1111/1471-0528.16313.

Ritchie, Jane, Jane Lewis, Carol McNaughton Nicholls, and Rachel Ormston, eds. 2013. *Qualitative Research Practice: A Guide for Social Science Students and Researchers*. 2nd ed. London: Sage.

Roberton, Timothy, Emily D. Carter, Victoria B. Chou, Angela R. Stegmuller, Bianca D. Jackson, Yvonne Tam, Talata Sawadogo-Lewis, and Neff Walker. 2020. "Early Estimates of the Indirect Effects of the COVID-19 Pandemic on Maternal and Child Mortality in Low-Income and Middle-Income Countries: A Modelling Study." *Lancet Global Health* 8 (7): e901–e908. https://doi.org/10.1016/s2214-109x(20)30229-1.

Sochas, Laura, Andrew Amos Channon, and Sara Nam. 2017. "Counting Indirect Crisis-Related Deaths in the Context of a Low-Resilience Health System: The Case of Maternal and Neonatal Health during the Ebola Epidemic in Sierra Leone." *Health Policy and Planning* 32 (3): iii32–iii39. https://doi.org/10.1093/heapol/czx108.

Stowe, Julia, Helen Smith, Kate Thurland, Mary E. Ramsay, Nick Andrews, and Shamez N. Ladhani. 2021. "Stillbirths during the COVID-19 Pandemic in England, April–June 2020." *JAMA* 325 (1): 86–87. https://doi.org/10.1001/jama.2020.21369.

Traviss, Gemma D., Robert. M. West, and Allan O. House. 2012. "Maternal Mental Health and its Association with Infant Growth at 6 Months in Ethnic Groups: Results from the Born-in-Bradford Birth Cohort Study." *PLoS One* 7 (2): e30707. https://doi.org/10.1371/journal.pone.0030707.

Knight, M., K. Bunch, N. Vousden, E. Morris, N. Simpson, C. Gale, et al. 2020. "Characteristics and Outcomes of Pregnant Women Admitted to Hospital with Confirmed SARS-CoV-2 Infection in UK: National Population Based Cohort Study." *BMJ* 369: m2107 https://doi.org/10.1136/bmj.m2107.

Vazquez-Vazquez, Adriana., Sarah Dib, Emeline Rougeaux, Jonathan C. Wells, and Mary S. Fewtrell. 2021. "The Impact of the COVID-19 Lockdown on the Experiences and Feeding Practices of New Mothers in the UK: Preliminary Data from the COVID-19 New Mum Study." *Appetite* 156: 104985. https://doi.org/10.1016/j.appet.2020.104985.

WHO (World Health Organization). 2018. *A Checklist for Pandemic Influenza Risk and Impact Management: Building Capacity for Pandemic Response*. Geneva: World Health Organization. https://apps.who.int/iris/bitstream/handle/10665/259884/9789241513623-eng.pdf?sequence=1.

WHO (World Health Organization). 2020a. "Companion of Choice During Labour and Childbirth for Improved Quality of Care: Evidence-to-Action Brief." https://apps.who.int/iris/bitstream/handle/10665/334151/WHO-SRH-20.13-eng.pdf.

WHO (World Health Organization). 2020b. "Pulse Survey on Continuity of Essential Health Services during the COVID-19 Pandemic: Interim Report, 27 August." September. https://apps.who.int/iris/rest/bitstreams/1297631/retrieve.

Williams, Candice, Rachel McKail, and Rukhsana Arshad. 2023. "'We Need To Be Heard. We Need To Be Seen': A Thematic Analysis of Black Maternal Experiences of Birthing and Postnatal Care in England within the Context of Covid-19." *Midwifery* 127: 103856.

Wu, Yanting, Chen Zhang, Han Liu, Chenchi Duan, Cheng Li, Jianxia Fan, Hong Li, et al. 2020. "Perinatal Depressive and Anxiety Symptoms of Pregnant Women during the Coronavirus Disease 2019 Outbreak in China." *American Journal of Obstetrics and Gynecology* 223 (2): 240.e1–240.e9. https://doi.org/10.1016/j.ajog.2020.05.009.

10 Women's Economic and Social Vulnerability to the Pandemic: Lessons from Bangladesh, Kenya, and Nigeria

Valerie Mueller, Nicole Wu, Atonu Rabbani, and Karen Grépin

Introduction

At the beginning of the COVID-19 pandemic, quantitative evidence showed that women around the world were especially vulnerable to the economic and social crises posed by school closures and lockdowns. Women increasingly were left to satisfy the growing demand for unpaid work at home (Del Boca et al. 2020; Agarwal 2021). Many exited the labor force (Seck et al. 2021; Kugler et al. 2023) and struggled with their mental health (Zamarro and Prados 2021; Xue and McMunn 2021). Patterns of economic precarity have also been associated with increased violence against women (Peterman et al. 2020; Agüero 2021). Although the narrative in earlier work focused mainly on the plight of women in high-income countries, an emerging literature in low-income countries painted a stark picture on the state of food insecurity (Josephson et al. 2021). Declines in income-generating activities affected not only the purchasing power of households but likely women's food consumption because of inequitable practices around food allocation (Kumar and Quisumbing 2013; D'Souza and Tandon 2019; Brown et al. 2021) and the weakening of supportive informal networks (Kumar et al. 2018).

In this chapter, we build on previous work in measuring the medium-term changes in women's outcomes to unravel which aspects of their well-being did and did not recover from initial losses. Specifically, we use data from women and men surveyed in Bangladesh, Kenya, and Nigeria at two time periods: an initial survey round conducted from November 2020 to January 21, 2021 (year 1) and another conducted during approximately the same months a year later in 2021–2022 (year 2). A disadvantage of the timing of our longitudinal study is that the first round of the survey took place months after the start of the COVID-19 pandemic. As such, we do not have prepandemic baseline data to really understand how the global implications of the pandemic influenced the well-being of our sample in terms of effects driven by inflation in market prices for staples or manufactured items. Our measure of recovery in essence compares the extent that beneficial outcomes were positively affected (or negative outcomes were reduced) in year 2 relative to year 1. We argue that comparisons of outcomes in years 1 and 2 still capture localized consequences of the pandemic, particularly in Kenya and Nigeria, where the enforcement of COVID-19 policies and the number of COVID-19 cases were rather low at the time of our first-round survey (Mueller et al. 2021; Mueller et al. 2022a). However, we are aware that comparisons of the outcomes over our study period might understate the magnitude of the localized effects in Bangladesh, where the number of infections was relatively high at the time of our first round (Abaluck et al. 2021) and school closures and lockdowns were quite stringent (Mueller et al. 2022a).

We also contribute to improvements in the measurement of equity-deserving groups and well-being metrics included in prior analysis (Egger et al. 2021; Josephson et al. 2021). First, we interviewed five hundred to eight hundred men in Bangladesh, Kenya, and Nigeria using the same survey instrument to differentiate whether the experience in losses was unique to women. Second, we included measures of well-being that have been ignored in the literature. Of particular interest is the integration of time use data to directly identify the extent to which women substituted paid for unpaid work as the burden of the demand for childcare and domestic services grew within the household. Time use data also allow us to capture the extent to which decisions related to time use led to women being deprived of sleep and leisure activities. We additionally measure how these habit-related changes coincided with changes in women's mental health. In addition to these contributions, we provide evidence of how women's employment and their household security, conflict, and food-related coping strategies were affected by the pandemic.

In what follows, we provide a brief overview of the longitudinal survey data collected in the three countries. We then describe our empirical methodology and reflect on changes in women's time use, employment, food insecurity and well-being amid the pandemic. We conclude with recommendations to policymakers based on our descriptive evidence.

Data

We collected three rounds of data during the pandemic in Bangladesh, Kenya, and Nigeria: round 1 (November 2020 to January 2021), round 2 (March and April 2021), and round 3 (November 2021 to January 2022). We only use data from rounds 1 and 3 in this analysis to provide inferences on the welfare consequences of COVID-19 over the course of a year and render comparisons within the same season or business cycle. The survey and human subject participation were reviewed locally by the National Health Research Ethics Committee of Nigeria in Nigeria (NHREC/01/01/2007), the Institutional Review Board of the BRAC James P. Grant School of Public Health at BRAC University in Bangladesh (IRB-13 October 20–043), and the Maseno University Ethics Review Committee in Kenya (MSU/DRPI/MUERC/00906/20). The study was also authorized by an institutional review board committee at Simon Fraser University in agreement with Arizona State University (FWA 00009102; IRB registration number IRB00000128) and the University of Hong Kong. The interviews were performed over mobile phones, and the sampling frame was achieved through the extension of a previous survey in Bangladesh and random digit dial methods in Kenya and Nigeria. The random digit dial approach consisted of purchasing numbers from third-party distributors and then randomly reaching a predetermined quota of men and women to create the national sample. We targeted roughly 1,200 women and 800 men at baseline. Respondents were surveyed if they met the following eligibility criteria: (1) they were at least eighteen years old; (2) they expressed a willingness to be resurveyed in the future and provided follow-up contact information (a phone number, their first name, and date of birth to verify their identity); and (3) they spoke one of the languages familiar to the enumerators on the team (e.g., English or Swahili in Kenya). Mueller et al. (2022a) provide greater detail on the survey design, the sample characteristics, and the national representativeness of data collected via random digit dial.

Survey Samples

The initial samples in round 1, in year 1, consisted of 1,822 individuals (914 men and 908 women) in Bangladesh, 2,038 individuals (744 men and 1,294 women) in Kenya, and 1,969 individuals (825 men and 1,144 women) in Nigeria. By round 3 (year 2), attrition was around 17 percent in Bangladesh, 33 percent in Kenya, and 35 percent in Nigeria. Our analysis relies on the responses of women and men who completed all three survey rounds: 1,547 individuals (793 men and 754 women) in Bangladesh, 1,367 individuals (524 men and 843 women) in Kenya, and 1,280 individuals (570 men and 710 women) in Nigeria. When comparing the attributes of the men and women who are included in our sample versus those who did not complete all three survey rounds, we find very few differences in Bangladesh. We find greater retention of educated (Nigeria) and older individuals (Bangladesh and Nigeria). Married women also tended to remain in the sample more frequently over time in Kenya and Nigeria. Our analysis used sampling weights in the construction of the summary statistics to resemble the national population more closely. In Kenya and Nigeria, the sampling weights provide an additional adjustment to correct for attrition. Mueller et al. (2022a) provide more information regarding the construction of sampling weights.

We provide a brief overview of the characteristics of our sample. The average ages of individuals in our samples at round 1 were forty-one and thirty-eight years old for men and women, respectively, in Bangladesh, twenty-eight years old for men and twenty-nine years old for women in Kenya, and thirty-eight and thirty-six years old for the men and women, respectively, in Nigeria. The percentages of men and women who had completed secondary education or higher at round 1 in Bangladesh are 32 percent and 28 percent, respectively; the percentages for those who had attended secondary education or higher at round 1 in Kenya are 88 percent and 85 percent, and in Nigeria, 91 percent and 88 percent. Thirty-eight percent of men and 36 percent of women were married in Kenya along with around 60 percent of both men and women in Nigeria, while the numbers are an astounding 93 percent of men and 72 percent of women in Bangladesh. The number of children (zero to eighteen years old) reported living in the respondents' households was around two for men and women in Bangladesh and Kenya, and three for men and women in Nigeria.

Outcomes Used in the Analysis

We summarize the main outcomes of interest in table 10.1 classified under themes of time use and employment, food insecurity, and well-being. We implemented a time use module where we asked individuals to recall how much time they had spent on the following activities in the last twenty-four hours: (1) school (including homework) and paid and unpaid work for wage labor or business; (2) getting health services for themselves or other household members; (3) cooking or other domestic work (including cleaning

Table 10.1
Summary of outcomes

Outcome variable	Description
Time use	
Work	Time used in the past 24 hours on school (including homework), work for salary or wages, or paid or unpaid work for business (farming, livestock, fishing, or nonagricultural activity)
Health	Time used in the past 24 hours on obtaining health services for self or other household members
Domestic work	Time used in the past 24 hours on cooking or other domestic work (including cleaning and fetching wood or water)
Child or adult care	Time used in the past 24 hours on unpaid care for children (including helping children with studies or schoolwork) or on unpaid care for adults (sick or elderly)
Shopping	Time used in the past 24 hours on shopping or buying goods
Travel	Time used in the past 24 hours on traveling and commuting
Social	Time used in past the 24 hours on religious activities or prayers and religious services, social activities, social media (Facebook, Instagram, Twitter), hobbies, or leisure (e.g., watching TV, listening to the radio, reading, exercise)
Sleeping	Time used in the past 24 hours on sleeping and resting or on personal care (bathing, grooming)
Eating	Time used in the past 24 hours on eating and drinking
Job and employment	
Employment	Individual worked for someone else or for themselves for pay for one or more hours in the past seven days
Food security	
Food-insecure	Household experienced not enough food or money to buy food in the past seven days
Mental health	
Probable anxiety	Has generalized anxiety disorder combined score greater than or equal to 3
Probable depression	Has patient health questionnaire combined score greater than or equal to 3
Security and conflict	
Feel secure	Household felt very or quite secure these days
No argument	Household had no argument in past six months
Argued once or twice	Household argued once or twice in past six months
Argued monthly or worse	Household argued monthly or more often in past six months
More conflict	Household had more conflict after COVID-19

and fetching wood or water); (4) unpaid care for children (including helping children with studies) or adults (sick or elderly); (5) shopping or buying goods; (6) traveling and commuting; (7) social activities (religious and social activities, social media, hobbies and leisure); (8) sleeping, resting, and personal care; and (9) eating and drinking. Minute increments were reported as fractions of hours. The responses from the time use module were used to create nine time use outcomes for the analysis. Employment is captured by a binary variable that assigns a value of 1 to those individuals who reported working at a paid job for at least one hour in the last seven days and 0 otherwise.

We also created outcomes to assess changes in food security, mental health, and security and conflict. We asked the respondents to first reflect on whether there were days (in the last week) when their household did not have enough food or money to buy food. We developed a binary outcome that assigned respondents a value of 1 for living in a food-insecure household if they answered yes to the question. We used questions from the mental health module of the survey questionnaire to develop two additional well-being indicators at the individual level. In the mental health module, we asked whether the individual over the last two weeks had been bothered by any of the following problems: (1) little interest or pleasure in doing things; (2) feeling down, depressed, or hopeless; (3) feeling nervous, anxious, or on edge; and (4) not being able to stop or control worrying. From the responses to these questions, we created two indicators: one of probable anxiety using the Generalized Anxiety Disorder (GAD)-2 screening tool and the other one demonstrating probable depression using the validated Patient Health Questionnaire (PHQ)-2 (Löwe et al. 2005; Kroenke et al. 2007; Plummer et al. 2016). Both assessments have possible scores ranging from 0 to 6. We created binary outcomes based on whether the values were greater than 3, which is indicative of probable anxiety and depression.

Finally, four outcomes were created based on the questions in the security and conflict module of the questionnaire. We created an outcome regarding whether the individual felt secure based on whether they indicated feeling very or quite secure these days compared to not very or not at all secure. We also borrowed a question designed by Peterman (2020) to examine the extent to which intrahousehold conflict had changed in Kenya and Nigeria:

> When people live together in the same household, they usually share both good and bad moments. And it is normal for people who live together to have arguments. How often in the last six months would you say that people in your household have argued or have had some sort of conflict among themselves?

Individuals could respond (1) never, (2) once or twice, (3) monthly, (4) weekly, (5) daily, (6) don't know, or (7) NA (for respondents who lived alone in the past six months). From the answers to this question, we created three binary indicators to reflect the proportion of individuals living in households without arguments, with arguments once or twice, and with more than one or two arguments. A final well-being indicator was constructed based on a follow-up question that asked the surveyed individuals to reflect on whether they believed conflicts within the household had increased since COVID-19. We created a binary outcome from those responses where a person received a value of 1 if they indicated that arguments were more frequent than before COVID-19 and a value of 0 if not.

Empirical Methodology and Results

In this section we describe how the outcomes changed for women in these three countries over the course of twelve months during the pandemic and then determine whether those changes were different from those experienced by men. Our approach was to first compare the mean values of the outcomes reported during the first and second years. We then discuss which differences are statistically meaningful, drawing from the results of t statistics reported in tables 10.2 and 10.3 that test whether those deviations are significant. Finally, we discuss whether these changes were uniquely experienced by women, also based on t tests that determine whether the change in the mean outcomes over time differ between the men and women respondents (tables 10.2 and 10.3). In what follows, we first present the results for time use and employment and then those for indicators of well-being (food security, mental health, and intrahousehold conflict).

Time Use and Employment

Figure 10.1 illustrates how the amount of time women spent on different activities changed over a one-year period during the pandemic. In table 10.2, we focus on the activities on which women spent most of their time: education and paid work, domestic work, social activities, sleeping, and childcare. The inclusion of childcare activities was motivated by the anticipated effects of disruptions in schooling schedules and barriers to childcare services during periodic curfews and lockdowns. To complement the time use outcomes, in table 10.2 we also summarize the changes in the proportion of women who obtained paid employment.

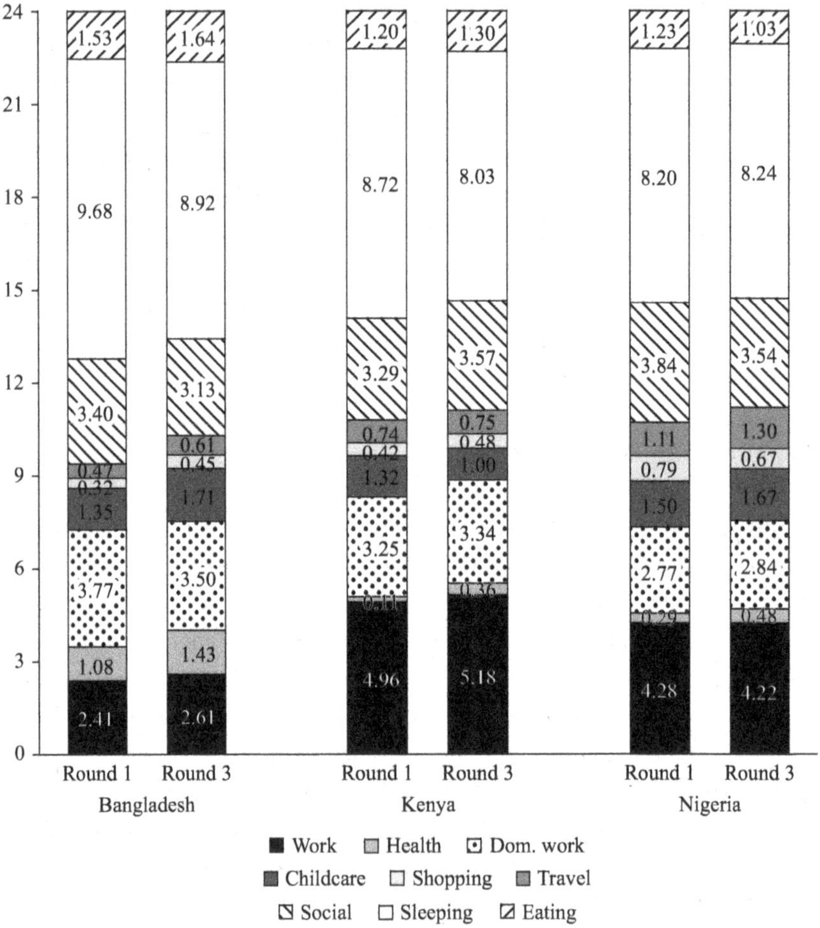

Figure 10.1
Changes in time use during the pandemic for women in Kenya, Nigeria, and Bangladesh.

The results indicate a slight increase in time spent in childcare over the year in Bangladesh (0.35 hours). Women in Kenya appeared to recover 0.32 hours devoted to childcare compared to round 1, which might have been affected by policies at the beginning of the pandemic (Mueller et al. 2022b). This decline seems to correspond with Kenyan women spending more time on paid work. For example, in year 2, women in Kenya report spending 0.32 hours less on childcare in a day and 0.22 hours more on paid work. However, the latter figure is not statistically meaningful. While the number of hours spent on domestic activities remained the same over the year for women in

Kenya and Nigeria, they declined by 0.27 hours for women in Bangladesh. In all three countries, there are no statistically meaningful changes in the number of hours women worked or in the proportion of women employed. Any gains in domestic work or childcare in Bangladesh and Kenya might have come at the expense of sleeping. Women in Bangladesh and Kenya spent 0.76 and 0.69 fewer hours sleeping, respectively, in comparison to round 1. Both of these trends could possibly correspond with a degradation in other aspects of well-being discussed in the next subsection.

Perhaps of broader interest is the extent to which these pandemic consequences were experienced by women alone. In columns 5, 10, and 15 of table 10.2, we compare the change in outcomes by gender and determine whether they are statistically meaningful according to the t test. Men and women faced the same experiences with respect to employment, with one exception: Bangladeshi men appeared to obtain fewer employment hours than women (0.47 hours).

Norms around childrearing and COVID-related policies might have created a unique burden for women in domestic and childcare activities. The declines in unpaid childcare as the pandemic progressed were entirely concentrated among women in Kenya. In the meantime, there was little change in the efforts devoted to domestic work and childcare in Nigeria. The analysis in Bangladesh illustrates that both men and women benefited over time in that they spent less time on domestic work, but they faced an increase in time spent on childcare. The magnitudes of these losses and gains in the various activities were no greater for women relative to men.

Food Insecurity and Well-Being

By the end of the study, we witnessed that food security improved for women relative to the first year (table 10.3). The proportion of women living in food-insecure households declined by 9 percent in Bangladesh, 13 percent in Kenya, and 8 percent in Nigeria. Our indicators at the household level show that men and women were progressing toward similar food security statuses. Changes in the tendency to be food-insecure do not statistically differ by gender according to the t tests reported in columns 5, 10, and 15 of table 10.3.

We next turn to the changes in women's mental health. Figure 10.2 breaks down the average anxiety (GAD-2) and depression (PHQ-2) scores calculated for women based on their survey responses at the start and end of the study period. All mental health scores worsened in the year 2 for women in Kenya

Table 10.2

Changes in time use and employment outcomes by gender in Kenya, Nigeria, and Bangladesh

	Bangladesh					Kenya					Nigeria				
	Women			Men		Women			Men		Women			Men	
	(1)	(2)	(3)	(4)	(5)	(6)	(7)	(8)	(9)	(10)	(11)	(12)	(13)	(14)	(15)
	R3	R1	R3-R1	R3-R1	(4)—(3)	R3	R1	R3-R1	R3-R1	(9)—(8)	R3	R1	R3-R1	R3-R1	(14)—(13)
	Mean/	Mean/	Mean/	Mean	Mean	Mean/	Mean/	Mean/	Mean	Mean	Mean/	Mean/	Mean/	Mean	Mean
	SE	SE	t test		t test	SE	SE	t test		t test	SE	SE	t test		t test
Time use															
Education and work	2.61 [0.13]	2.41 [0.13]	0.20	−0.43**	−0.63***	5.18 [0.28]	4.96 [0.28]	0.22	1.01**	0.79	4.22 [0.19]	4.28 [0.20]	−0.05	0.48*	0.53
Domestic work	3.50 [0.08]	3.77 [0.09]	−0.27**	−0.39***	−0.12	3.34 [0.13]	3.25 [0.13]	0.09	−0.11	−0.20	2.84 [0.10]	2.77 [0.10]	0.07	0.00	−0.07
Unpaid childcare	1.71 [0.06]	1.35 [0.08]	0.35***	0.36***	0.01	1.00 [0.08]	1.32 [0.11]	−0.32**	0.07	0.39*	1.67 [0.10]	1.50 [0.10]	0.17	−0.01	−0.18
Social activities	3.13 [0.08]	3.40 [0.09]	−0.27**	0.11	0.37***	3.57 [0.14]	3.29 [0.15]	0.28	−0.49*	−0.77**	3.54 [0.12]	3.84 [0.14]	−0.30	−0.45**	−0.16
Sleeping	8.92 [0.08]	9.68 [0.08]	−0.76***	−0.44***	0.31**	8.03 [0.15]	8.72 [0.15]	−0.69***	−1.13***	−0.44	8.24 [0.15]	8.20 [0.17]	0.04	0.23	0.19
Employment															
Paid work	0.15 [0.02]	0.13 [0.02]	0.02	0.01	−0.01	0.58 [0.03]	0.50 [0.03]	0.08	0.06	−0.02	0.55 [0.03]	0.57 [0.03]	−0.01	−0.01	−0.00
N	754	754		793		843	843		524		710	710		570	

Note: Standard errors in brackets. *** $p<0.01$, ** $p<0.05$, * $p<0.1$. The t tests in columns 3, 8, and 13 use the sampling weights in the respective rounds (e.g. baseline in R1 and R3 weights accounting for attrition in R3). Similarly, the corresponding t tests in columns 4, 9, and 14 for the male sample use the sampling weights in the respective rounds. The t statistics presented in columns 5, 10, and 15 are based on calculations that compare the change in outcomes by gender, where the sampling weights applied are only for R3.

Table 10.3
Changes in food insecurity and well-being outcomes by gender in Kenya, Nigeria, and Bangladesh

	Bangladesh					Kenya					Nigeria				
	Women			Men		Women			Men		Women			Men	
	(1)	(2)	(3)	(4)	(5)	(6)	(7)	(8)	(9)	(10)	(11)	(12)	(13)	(14)	(15)
	R3	R1	R3-R1	R3-R1	(4)—(3)	R3	R1	R3-R1	R3-R1	(9)—(8)	R3	R1	R3-R1	R3-R1	(14)—(13)
	Mean/ SE	Mean/ SE	Mean/ t test	Mean	Mean t test	Mean/ SE	Mean/ SE	Mean/ t test	Mean	Mean t test	Mean/ SE	Mean/ SE	Mean/ t test	Mean	Mean t test
Food security															
Household	0.19	0.28	−0.09***	−0.13***	−0.03	0.46	0.60	−0.13***	−0.11*	0.02	0.42	0.51	−0.08**	−0.09**	−0.01
food-insecure	[0.02]	[0.02]				[0.03]	[0.03]				[0.03]	[0.03]			
N	754	754		793		843	843		524		710	710		570	
Mental health															
Probable anxiety	0.03	0.13	−0.10***	−0.07***	0.03	0.20	0.06	0.14***	0.11***	−0.03	0.21	0.11	0.10***	0.09***	−0.01
	[0.01]	[0.02]				[0.03]	[0.01]				[0.02]	[0.02]			
Probable	0.36	0.43	−0.07**	−0.03	0.05	0.24	0.06	0.18***	0.11***	−0.07*	0.27	0.15	0.13***	0.10***	−0.03
depression	[0.02]	[0.02]				[0.03]	[0.01]				[0.02]	[0.02]			
N	754	754		793		843	843		524		710	710		570	
Security and conflict															
Feel secure	0.88	0.57	0.32***	0.39***	0.08**	0.83	0.73	0.10***	0.14***	0.03	0.70	0.65	0.05	0.07**	0.02
	[0.01]	[0.02]				[0.03]	[0.03]				[0.02]	[0.03]			
N	754	754		792		843	843		524		710	710		570	
Household had no						0.39	0.31	0.08	0.15**	0.07	0.41	0.44	−0.03	−0.01	0.02
arguments						[0.04]	[0.03]				[0.03]	[0.03]			
Household argued						0.28	0.32	−0.04	−0.02	0.01	0.30	0.33	−0.03	−0.10**	−0.07
once or twice						[0.03]	[0.03]				[0.03]	[0.03]			
Household argued monthly						0.33	0.37	−0.04	−0.12*	−0.08	0.29	0.23	0.06*	0.11***	0.04
or more						[0.03]	[0.03]				[0.02]	[0.02]			
N						738	738		393		614	614		447	
More conflict since	0.13	0.33	−0.20***	−0.14***	0.06	0.66	0.53	0.13***	−0.00	−0.14*	0.33	0.47	−0.15***	−0.14***	0.01
COVID-19	[0.02]	[0.03]				[0.03]	[0.03]				[0.03]	[0.03]			
N	590	590		655		782	782		444		589	589		455	

Note: Standard errors in brackets. *** $p<0.01$, ** $p<0.05$, * $p<0.1$. The t tests in columns 3, 8, and 13 use the sampling weights in the respective rounds (e.g., baseline in R1 and R3 weights accounting for attrition in R3). Similarly, the corresponding t tests in columns 4, 9, and 14 for the men's sample use the sampling weights in the respective rounds. The t statistics presented in columns 5, 10, and 15 are based on calculations that compare the change in outcomes by gender, where the sampling weights applied are only for R3.

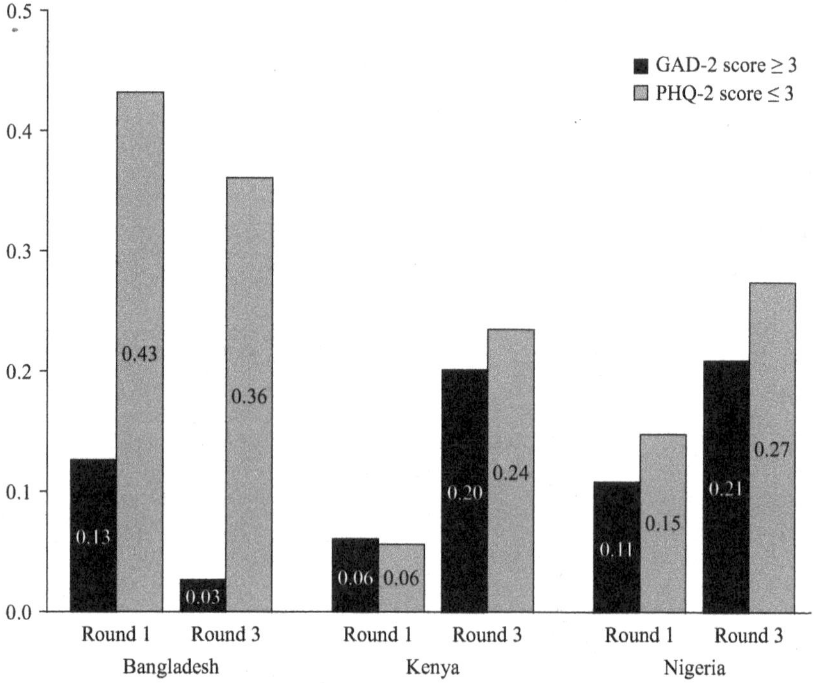

Figure 10.2
Changes in mental health status during the pandemic for women in Kenya, Nigeria, and Bangladesh.

and Nigeria. The proportion of women with probable anxiety and depression declined in year 2 for women in Bangladesh. The t statistics in columns 3, 8, and 13 in table 10.3 illustrate that the differences portrayed in figure 10.2 are statistically significant according to the t tests. The mental health figures illustrate that there are no gendered differences in the changes in anxiety. The increase in the proportion of women who became depressed by year 2 in Kenya was 18 percent, which is 7 percent more than the growth in depression among men. The short-term consequences on food insecurity (Mueller et al. 2022a) and time use and employment (Mueller et al. 2022b) may have created a mental toll on women in the long term in Kenya. Similarly, disruptions in sleeping patterns among Kenyan women may have exacerbated their psychological stress, according to the recent body of COVID-19 literature (Alimoradi et al. 2021; Alimoradi 2022).

A final set of well-being indicators considered in the analysis comprised metrics related to security and conflict. With the exception of women in Nigeria, women reported feeling more secure during the second survey round relative to the first year of the pandemic. Feelings were relatively similar across genders in Kenya. In Kenya, women reported having fewer arguments at home as time went on, but a greater number reported having more conflicts than prior to COVID-19. These sentiments were not consistent with those of men. In Bangladesh, a higher proportion of men, relative to women, felt more secure at the end of the study. Perhaps conflicts within the household might additionally contribute to the disruptions in sleeping patterns and the overall toll on women's mental health.

The reports on security and conflict from respondents in Nigeria and Bangladesh offer a few puzzling results. For example, both men and women in Nigeria consistently reported arguing more at the end of the study period relative to round 1, but less than prior to COVID-19. In Bangladesh, both men and women report having fewer arguments than before COVID-19. One potential explanation for the inconsistent information is that measurement error may increase on self-reported information as the recall period increases over time. Here, the recall period refers to since COVID-19, a period that grew by year 2. Another possible rationale may be that there are other temporal dimensions that contribute to tension in the household that we failed to capture in this study. This is one drawback in having to conduct a phone interview using a short survey instrument and not having interviewed the respondents prior to COVID-19. Not only do we lack information about the well-being of the respondents prior to COVID-19 to have an objective measure prior to the pandemic, but we had to trade off asking detailed questions pertaining to well-being with other crucial questions related to the political, economic, and social factors that have the potential to exacerbate tensions with the household prior to the study.

Conclusion

Gendered norms around the allocation of unpaid and paid work stymie women's economic empowerment and well-being globally. The health crisis appears to have exacerbated these gender inequities. Women were expected to bear the increased burden of domestic work and childcare driven by school closures and mobility restrictions, while their ability to outsource these activities through formal and informal channels became limited. These features of the pandemic reinforced an already low rate of labor force participation among women. As norms constrain women's economic potential in the long term, prioritizing campaigns that shift perspectives around caregiving and domestic work may reduce gender inequities and promote economic growth in all contexts (Hsieh et al. 2019).

The descriptive evidence suggests that the type of programs required to address inequities in the short term will vary by context and depend on an alliance of social protection policies, educational reforms, and health interventions (Hidrobo et al. 2020). While the growing evidence in relation to the suspension of COVID-19 policies has demonstrated that relaxation has allowed children to access their meals at school (Abay et al. 2021) and allowed other household members to spend more time at work (Mueller et al. 2022b), observed declines in mental health, disruptions in sleeping patterns, and the rise in arguments within the household continued. Power relations may operate to reproduce inequality but also challenge it at times. Kenyan women were able to recover the time spent on unpaid work to increase employment. Fewer changes were observed among women in Nigeria. In the meantime, men and women faced similar disruptions in their employment in Bangladesh, yet recovery was worse for men than women. Improvements among women coincided with more harmonious relations in the household. This suggests that existing health institutions should be strengthened in these countries to incorporate affordable psychological services for mothers and couples (Ajayi et al. 2021). Ajayi et al. (2021) note innovative ways of delivering these services through tele-consulting or leveraging the existing network of community health workers.

Childcare constraints may continue to be responsible for inequities in labor force participation that have existed since before COVID-19 and are ongoing today (Bidisha et al. 2022). Governments should expand early childhood educational programs to reduce the burden of childcare on women (Tang et al. 2021). This can reduce the variability in access that results from a reliance on informal childcare networks and efficiently target the most vulnerable groups of women, such as mothers of young children from liquidity-constrained households.

References

Abaluck, Jason, Laura H. Kwong, Ashley Styczynski, Ashraful Haque, Alamgir Kabir, Ellen Bates-Jefferys, Emily Crawford, et al. 2021. "Impact of Community Masking on COVID-19: A Cluster-Randomized Trial in Bangladesh." *Science* 375 (6577): eabi9069. https://doi.org/10.1126/science.abi9069.

Abay, Kibrom A., Mulubrhan Amare, Luca Tiberti, and Kwaw S. Andam. 2021. "COVID-19 Induced Disruptions of School Feeding Services Exacerbate Food Insecurity in Nigeria." *Journal of Nutrition* 151 (8): 2245–2254. https://doi.org/10.1093/jn/nxab100.

Agarwal, Bina. 2021. "Livelihoods in COVID Times: Gendered Perils and New Pathways in India." *World Development* 139: 105312. https://doi.org/10.1016/j.worlddev.2020.105312.

Agüero, Jorge M. 2021. "COVID-19 and the Rise of Intimate Partner Violence." *World Development* 137: 105217. https://doi.org/10.1016/j.worlddev.2020.105217.

Ajayi, Kobi V., Elizabeth Wachira, Obasanjo Afolabi Bolarinwa, and Beulah D. Suleman. 2021. "Maternal Mental Health in Africa during the COVID-19 Pandemic: A Neglected Global Health Issue." *Epidemiology and Health* 43: e2021078. https://doi.org/10.4178/epih.e2021078.

Alimoradi, Zainab, Fatemeh Abdi, David Gozal, and Amir H. Pakpour. 2022. "Estimation of Sleep Problems among Pregnant Women during COVID-19 Pandemic: A Systematic Review and Meta-Analysis." *BMJ Open* 12 (4): e056044. https://doi.org/10.1136/bmjopen-2021-056044.

Alimoradi, Zainab, Anders Broström, Hector W. H. Tsang, Mark D. Griffiths, Shahab Haghayegh, Maurice M. Ohayon, Chung-Ying Lin, and Amir H. Pakpour. 2021. "Sleep Problems during COVID-19 Pandemic and Its' Association to Psychological Distress: A Systematic Review and Meta-Analysis." *EClinicalMedicine* 36: 100916. https://doi.org/10.1016/j.eclinm.2021.100916.

Bidisha, Sayema Haque, Avinno Faruk, and Tanveer Mahmood. 2022. "How Are Women Faring in the Bangladeshi Labour Market? Evidence from Labour Force Survey Data." *South Asia Economic Journal* 23 (2): 201–227. https://doi.org/10.1177/13915614221108564.

Brown, Caitlin, Rossella Calvi, and Jacob Penglase. 2021. "Sharing the Pie: An Analysis of Undernutrition and Individual Consumption in Bangladesh." *Journal of Public Economics* 200: 104460. https://doi.org/10.1016/j.jpubeco.2021.104460.

Del Boca, Daniela, Noemi Oggero, Paola Profeta, and Maria Cristina Rossi. 2020. "Women's and Men's Work, Housework and Childcare, Before and During COVID-19." *Review of Economics of the Household* 18: 1001–1017. https://www.iza.org/publications/dp/13409/womens-work-housework-and-childcare-before-and-during-covid-19.

D'Souza, Anna, and Sharad Tandon 2019. "Intrahousehold Nutritional Inequities in Rural Bangladesh." *Economic Development and Cultural Change* 67 (3): 625–657. https://doi.org/10.1086/698311.

Egger, Dennis, Edward Miguel, Shana S. Warren, Ashish Shenoy, Elliott Collins, Dean Karlan, Doug Parkerson, et al. 2021. "Falling Living Standards during the COVID-19 Crisis: Quantitative Evidence from Nine Developing Countries." *Science Advances* 7 (6): eabe0997. https:// doi.org/10.1126/sciadv.abe0997.

Hidrobo, Melissa, Neha Kumar, Tia Palermo, Amber Peterman, and Shalini Roy. 2020. "Gender-Sensitive Social Protection: A Critical Component of the COVID-19 Response in Low- and Middle-Income Countries." International Food Policy Research Institute (IFPRI) Issue Brief, April. https://doi.org/10.2499/9780896293793.

Hsieh, Chang-Tai, Erik Hurst, Charles I. Jones, and Peter J. Klenow. 2019. "The Allocation of Talent and Economic Growth." *Econometrica* 87 (5): 1439–1474. https:// doi.org/10.3982/ECTA11427.

Josephson, Anna, Talip Kilic, and Jeffrey D. Michler. 2021. "Socioeconomic Impacts of COVID-19 in Low-Income Countries." *Nature Human Behavior* 5 (5): 557–565. https://doi.org/10.1038/s41562-021-01096-7.

Kroenke, Kurt, Robert L. Spitzer, Janet B. W. Williams, Patrick O. Monahan, and Bernd Löwe. 2007. "Anxiety Disorders in Primary Care: Prevalence, Impairment, Comorbidity, and Detection." *Annals of Internal Medicine* 146 (5): 317–325. https:// doi.org/10.7326/0003-4819-146-5-200703060-00004.

Kugler, Maurice, Mariana Viollaz, Daniel Duque, Isis Gaddis, David Newhouse, Amparo Palacios-Lopez, and Michael Weber. 2023. "How Did the COVID-19 Crisis Affect Different Types of Workers in the Developing World?" *World Development* 170: 106331.

Kumar, Neha, and Agnes R. Quisumbing 2013. "Gendered Impacts of the 2007–2008 Food Price Crisis: Evidence Using Panel Data from Rural Ethiopia." *Food Policy* 38: 11–22. https://doi.org/10.1016/j.foodpol.2012.10.002.

Kumar, Neha, Samuel Scott, Purnima Menon, Samyuktha Kannan, Kenda Cunningham, Parul Tyagi, Gargi Wable, Kalyani Raghunathan, and Agnes Quisumbing. 2018. "Pathways from Women's Group-Based Programs to Nutrition Change in South Asia: A Conceptual Framework and Literature Review." *Global Food Security* 17: 172–185. https://doi.org/10.1016/j.gfs.2017.11.002.

Löwe, Bernd, Kurt Kroenke, and Kerstin Gräfe. 2005. "Detecting and Monitoring Depression with a Two-Item Questionnaire (PHQ-2)." *Journal of Psychosomatic Research* 58 (2): 163–171. https://doi.org/10.1016/j.jpsychores.2004.09.006.

Mueller, Valerie, Karen A. Grépin, Atonu Rabbani, Bianca Navia, Anne S. W. Ngunjiri, and Nicole Wu. 2022a. "Food Insecurity and COVID-19 Risk in Low- and

Middle-Income Countries." *Applied Economic Perspectives and Policy* 44 (1): 92–109. https://doi.org/10.1002/aepp.13200.

Mueller, Valerie, Karen A. Grépin, Atonu Rabbani, Anne Ngunjiri, Amy Oyekunle, and Clare Wenham. 2022b. "Domestic Burden amid COVID-19 and Women's Mental Health in Middle-Income Africa." Paper presented at the Population Association Conference of America in Atlanta, Georgia on April 8, 2022.

Peterman, Amber, Alina Potts, Megan O'Donnell, Kelly Thompson, Niyati Shah, Sabine Oertelt-Prigione, and Nicole van Gelder. 2020. "Pandemics and Violence against Women and Children." *Center for Global Development*, April. https://www.cgdev.org/sites/default/files/pandemics-and-vawg-april2.pdf.

Plummer, Faye, Laura Manea, Dominic Trepel, and Dean McMillan. 2016. "Screening for Anxiety Disorders with the GAD-7 and GAD-2: A Systematic Review and Diagnostic Metaanalysis." *General Hospital Psychiatry* 39: 24–31. https://doi.org/10.1016/j.genhosppsych.2015.11.005.

Seck, Papa A., Jessamyn O. Encarnacion, Cecilia Tinonin, and Sara Duerto-Valero. 2021. "Gendered Impacts of COVID-19 in Asia and the Pacific: Early Evidence on Deepening Socioeconomic Inequalities in Paid and Unpaid Work." *Feminist Economics* 27 (1–2): 117–132. https://doi.org/10.1080/13545701.2021.1876905.

Tang, Vincent, Aroa Santiago, Zohra Khan, David Amaglobeli, Esuna Dugarova, Katherine Gifford, Laura Gores, et al. 2021. "Gender Equality and COVID-19: Policies and Institutions for Mitigating the Crisis." International Monetary Fund. https://www.imf.org/-/media/Files/Publications/covid19-special-notes/en-special-series-on-covid-19-gender-equality-and-covid-19.ashx.

Xue, Baowen, and Anne McMunn. 2021. "Gender Differences in Unpaid Care Work and Psychological Distress in the UK COVID-19 Lockdown." *PLoS One* 16 (3): e0247959. https://doi.org/10.1371/journal.pone.0247959.

Zamarro, Gema, and María J. Prados. 2021. "Gender Differences in Couples' Division of Childcare, Work and Mental Health During COVID-19." *Review of Economics of the Household* 19: 11–40. https://doi.org/10.1007/s11150-020-09534-7.

11 Gender-Responsive Pandemic Planning

Heang-Lee Tan, Kate Hawkins, Erica Rosser, Julia Smith,
Clare Wenham, and Rosemary Morgan

Introduction

As the previous chapters in this book demonstrate, the COVID-19 pandemic has been particularly brutal for women and other marginalized groups. The pandemic had both primary and secondary impacts. Primary impacts are immediate, direct impacts, such as COVID-19 infections, deaths, and related illnesses, while secondary impacts are long-term social, economic, and non-COVID-19 health impacts (Tan et al. 2021). Although some primary impacts have been greater among men—for example, more men have contracted and died from COVID-19—measures to reduce COVID-19 infections and deaths, such as lockdowns and school closures, have led to greater secondary impacts among women and other marginalized groups. Here, we focus specifically on the experiences of women, particularly those most likely to experience gender inequality alongside and in relation to other inequities. The recurring theme is that women—particularly those who are poor and from marginalized groups—shouldered the brunt of the secondary impacts of the pandemic and bore primary responsibility for managing the measures to limit disease transmission. Despite the structural barriers that disadvantage specific groups of women in many of the contexts highlighted thus far, it is crucial to remember that governments *can* enact policy interventions to minimize these impacts on those women most affected. Gender-responsive pandemic plans take into account the disproportionate impact of pandemics on groups of marginalized women by using an intersectional gender lens in planning, data collection, response, and recovery. In this way, interventions can mitigate the gendered economic, social, and health impacts of a pandemic (Rosser et al. 2021).

In this chapter, we explore how gender-responsive pandemic plans can mitigate the secondary impacts of the pandemic by shining a spotlight on the following areas: livelihoods and social protection, care work, the health workforce, mental health, essential health services, gender-based violence, education, and participation in decision-making. Across these areas, we offer snapshots of measures adopted by governments around the world and lessons on how to bring greater equality to pandemic policies. As our discussion on gender-responsive pandemic plans would be incomplete without addressing the very real issue of political prioritization, we also discuss what factors enable gender equity to be prioritized in the pandemic response.

Gender-Responsive Pandemic Planning

A gender-responsive pandemic plan considers the needs of women, men, and gender minorities when developing policies to prevent, detect, respond to, and recover from a pandemic, as well as the range of intersectional challenges they face. This begins with a clear assessment of gender-related knowledge, gender-related gaps, and areas for gender-based development. When developing a gender-responsive pandemic plan, a multisectoral, iterative, and dynamic approach is key to responding to the evolution of the outbreak and virus. Intersectional disaggregated data must be gathered at all stages of the pandemic life cycle, and this data must be analyzed and used to inform and implement an evidence-based pandemic plan (Figure 11.1).

Before a pandemic Lessons from previous health emergencies, as well as context-specific information within a jurisdiction, should inform the preparedness plan and associated budgeting. Gender-responsive budgeting allows for allocation and prioritization of resources to programs and initiatives to mitigate the impact of a health emergency on the most vulnerable, including protocols on how funding will be available and to whom and when. The multisectoral landscape of actors potentially involved in pandemic response should develop commitments about what they will do should an emergency arise and about methods to reduce gender inequalities at every stage of pandemic management. This landscape of actors must include those who represent the target group for interventions (i.e., women, gender minorities, and other marginalized groups) as well as meaningful collaboration and work with gender experts and organizations focused on gender equality.

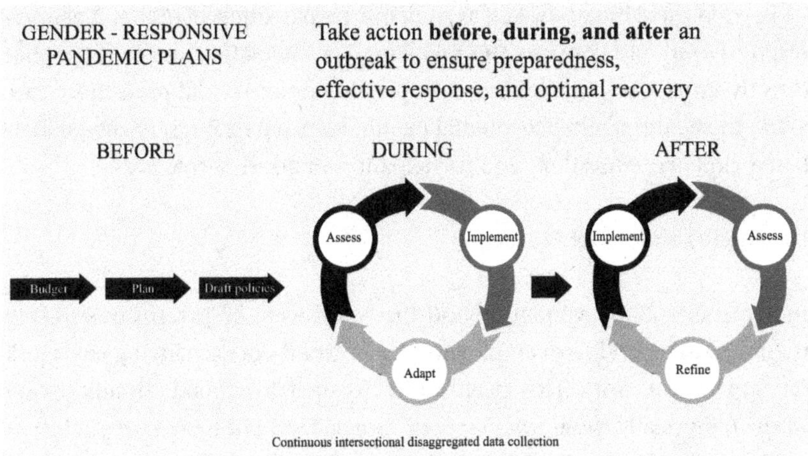

Figure 11.1
Continuous intersectional disaggregated data collection for gender responsive pandemic planning (Rosser et al. 2021).

During a pandemic A government that has prepared to mitigate the secondary gendered effects of a pandemic (i.e., by following the "before" steps) is well positioned to act decisively on the emergence of a pathogen. Rapid gender-based analysis in the initial phase of the epidemic can determine whether all eventualities have been accounted for or if the outbreak in question poses differential effects for particular groups owing to transmission patterns. This can then lead to implementation strategies to mitigate gendered effects during transmission, depending on the epidemiological context. Multisectoral, reflective collaboration at this stage is vital to take a whole-of-society approach and to build and improve the strategies implemented in light of new gender-disaggregated data and advice from affected groups.

After a pandemic Meaningful reconstruction and recovery depend on maintaining support across society and particularly for the most vulnerable. Action reviews at multiple stages can identify whether recovery strategies have served the needs of people of all genders, and policies can then be improved accordingly. Documentation can ensure that broader learnings can be incorporated into more mainstream social and health policies (Rosser et al. 2021).

Beyond these broad strokes, a pandemic preparedness plan that is gender-responsive should consider the following key thematic areas as those that directly impact marginalized groups: livelihoods and social protection, care work, the health workforce, mental health, essential health services, gender-based violence, education, and participation in decision-making.

Livelihoods and Social Protection

In September 2021, women around the world were 27 percent more likely than men to report loss of employment, many of them exchanging paid work for unpaid care work (Flor et al. 2022). As their livelihoods shrank, many women, especially those who are poor, struggled to put food on the table, as evidenced in chapter 3, on Bangladesh, in this volume. In many countries, women were also more likely to work in the informal sector and to hold precarious jobs without social security—as highlighted in chapters 7, 4, and 5, on Hong Kong, Brazil, and Canada, respectively—which made women even more vulnerable to job loss during the crisis.

One response to the economic fallout of the pandemic is cash transfer programs. However, surveys across forty-five countries found that only 10 percent of women surveyed received government cash transfers during the first year of the pandemic, compared to 16 percent of men (UN Women 2021b). Gender-blind cash transfers aimed at households often do not reach women due to gendered power relations within families. In Malaysia, according to Joanne M. Wong, head of programs at the Women's Aid Organisation, the country's largest domestic violence service provider, some survivors whom it served did not receive government cash transfers, which were disbursed to households, because their husbands were the first household members to apply for the funds (Joanne M. Wong, personal communication). In some instances, abusive husbands retaliated when their partners successfully applied for the funds before they did, leading to an escalation in domestic violence (Joanne M. Wong, personal communication). Designers of cash transfer programs must be sensitive to gendered power relations within the household and include measures to facilitate women's access to funds.

An example of a cash transfer program that prioritized women and informal workers is *Auxílio Emergencial* (Emergency Aid) in Brazil, which was introduced in April 2020 to supplement the existing *Bolsa Familia* (Family Purse) cash transfer program (Staab et al. 2022). Those eligible for *Auxílio Emergencial* included existing *Bolsa Familia* recipients, as well as self-employed or informal workers who were affected by COVID-19 (Gentilini et al. 2022). Single mothers received twice the benefits (1,200 Brazilian *reals* or USD 232 per month) for the first nine months of the program (Staab et al. 2022).

As countries move toward digital cash transfers, there is a corresponding need to increase women's access to the internet, phones, computers, and bank accounts to ensure that women, particularly those of low socioeconomic status, are not excluded from receiving these transfers. In 2021, across low- and middle-income countries, women were 16 percent less likely to use mobile internet and 18 percent less likely to own a smartphone compared to men (Shanahan 2022). Women are also less likely to have bank accounts. In 2021, only 68 percent of women age fifteen and above in low- and middle-income countries had bank accounts, compared to 74 percent of their male counterparts (World Bank 2021b, 2021a). Financial and digital inclusion would not only help women access digital cash transfers but would also enable them to participate in e-commerce, which has become even more important since the pandemic began (UNCTAD 2021).

Care Work

During the initial months of the pandemic, as schools and childcare centers shut their doors and household members fell ill, caregiving responsibilities at home piled high. Due to inequitable gender roles and norms, the bulk of caregiving responsibilities fell on women's shoulders, with just a fraction of men stepping up to share these responsibilities equally. In 2020, across twenty-five OECD countries, mothers were nearly three times more likely than fathers to shoulder most or all of the additional caregiving responsibilities due to school or childcare center closures (OECD 2021)—trends that are also reflected in the diverse case studies featured in this book. As demonstrated in the chapters here, as well as other research, these increased care burdens cost women economic, employment, and educational opportunities as well as increasing stress and reducing time for social and political engagement.

A handful of countries recognized the added care burden created by the pandemic and introduced policies to mitigate associated costs. In Argentina, for example, parents were allowed excused absences from work for childcare reasons during school closures, and these arrangements continued when schools reopened with shorter hours (Staab et al. 2022). Another measure to support families is cash-for-care programs. In Germany, for example, employees with children below the age of twelve or with a disability were eligible for income loss compensation for up to six weeks at two-thirds of their usual income, up to a monthly maximum of EUR 2,016 (USD 2,303) (Staab et al. 2022). Such programs helped caregivers make up for lost income due to increased caregiving responsibilities during the pandemic. However, a major limitation of such policies is that they only benefit those in formal employment.

While family leave and cash-for-care policies can reduce conflicts between unpaid care work and paid work time for those in formal employment, they can also reinforce the norm that caregiving is women's responsibility. Such initiatives need to also target men and encourage them to play their part in caregiving. For example, parental leave policies that designate a portion of leave for fathers, on a use-it-or-lose-it basis, may increase uptake of parental leave by men (Janta and Steward 2019). Pandemic care policies might also include such incentives.

Other governments have focused on addressing the underlying weaknesses in the care economy that have been exposed by the pandemic. The Canadian government, for example, introduced a new nationwide early learning and childcare strategy in 2021 (Department of Finance Canada 2021). Under the program, the federal government pledged to invest CAD (Canadian dollars) 30 billion over five years to reduce the cost and increase the accessibility of childcare, aiming to achieve an average cost of CAD 10 per day per child by 2026 (Department of Finance Canada 2021). The government has noted that the program would benefit both families and the economy, as it would create new caregiving jobs and help women stay in the workforce. It is estimated that the program could increase the country's gross domestic product by up to 1.2 percent over the next two decades (Department of Finance Canada 2021). In addition, a strong childcare system would ensure that the country is better prepared to deal with shocks to the care economy in the event of future health crises.

Health Workforce

Women make up 70 percent of health workers worldwide and tend to occupy lower-paid, frontline positions, where racialized and migrant women are particularly overrepresented. As chapters 4, 6, and 8, from Brazil, China, and Kenya, respectively, demonstrate, this work is essential to pandemic responses. However, many women healthcare workers do not have adequate access to personal protective equipment (PPE), training, or other necessities to keep themselves and those they care for safe during infectious disease outbreaks. For example, standard PPE is often made to fit men's, not women's, bodies. Due to the overload of both paid and unpaid care responsibilities during the COVID-19 pandemic, many women healthcare workers faced extreme moral distress and related burnout (Smith et al. 2022). By working on the front lines of the response, healthcare workers are also at risk of stigma and abuse, particularly healthcare workers from racial and other minority groups (Wenham et al. 2022).

To support healthcare workers, thirty-one countries provided salary top-ups or one-off bonuses to healthcare workers during the pandemic (Staab et al. 2022). However, only nine salary top-up programs specifically targeted lower-paid healthcare workers (Staab et al. 2022). To ensure equity, financial compensation programs must cover healthcare workers in lower-paid or lower-status positions, such as midwives, care workers, community health workers, and cleaning and support staff. In Cuba, for example, the government gave an additional 250 Cuban pesos (~USD 10) per month to hospital support staff involved in food service, laundry, and sanitation, and about 78 percent of those who received this salary top-up were women (UNDP 2022).

In addition to providing compensation, health systems can also meet healthcare workers' basic needs by providing adequate PPE, training, childcare, meals, transportation, onsite rest spaces, and alternative housing arrangements for those who are isolating from family (David et al. 2022). In countries such as Costa Rica, Guyana, Japan, South Korea, and Singapore, for example, emergency childcare was provided to essential workers (Staab et al. 2022). Meeting healthcare workers' basic needs helps reduce workplace stressors, which in turn protects their mental health and well-being (David et al. 2022). Notably, a study in China found that healthcare workers were less inclined to engage in mental health programs when their basic needs had yet to be met (David et al. 2022).

In addition, women healthcare workers must be given opportunities to participate in decision-making and to provide input on institutional pandemic policies (Morgan et al. 2022). Input from frontline health workers is critical, as they have direct knowledge of patient needs as well as what measures are feasible and practical in a crisis. Involving healthcare workers in decision-making harnesses their experiential expertise and contributions to the pandemic response and increases their sense of control and autonomy in a situation that is rife with uncertainty.

Mental Health

Rates of anxiety and depression skyrocketed around the world as people and their communities reeled from the trauma of the pandemic (COVID-19 Mental Disorders Collaborators 2021). For women, the mental health toll was greater, possibly because they were more likely to lose jobs, shoulder heavier caregiving responsibilities, and face violence at home (COVID-19 Mental Disorders Collaborators 2021). Indeed, multiple chapters in this book indicate that both financial insecurity and increased unpaid care contributed to ongoing poor mental health. It is estimated that the pandemic contributed to 87.3 million additional cases of anxiety disorder and major depressive disorder among women globally, compared to 42.1 million additional cases of these disorders among men (COVID-19 Mental Disorders Collaborators 2021).

In 2016, countries around the world spent less than 2 percent of their healthcare budget, on average, on mental health (The Lancet Global Health 2020; World Health Organization 2018). Moreover, in 27 percent of 169 countries, care and treatment for mental health disorders were excluded from national health insurance or reimbursement schemes, forcing many people to pay out-of-pocket for mental health services (The Lancet Global Health 2020; World Health Organization 2018). As countries chart a path of recovery from the pandemic, this trend should be reversed, with increased prioritization and investment in mental health.

There is also a need to train more mental health providers, as the shortage of qualified providers is a key factor limiting the availability of mental health services. Mental health training should incorporate culturally appropriate, trauma-informed care, given the trauma that many communities faced during the pandemic. Trauma-informed care recognizes the prevalence and impact of trauma and seeks to avoid retraumatization (Agency for Clinical Innovation n.d.). Understandably, increasing the number of mental health providers is a long-term endeavor, and in the short term, countries can scale up mental health services by exploring innovative digital approaches, such as mental health apps. However, digital resources and services cannot completely replace in-person services, as the former may not be accessible to everyone.

Disruptions in Essential Health Services

During the pandemic, essential health services for women were disrupted due to both supply and demand factors, as highlighted in the UK case study in chapter 10. Research across thirty-nine low- and middle-income countries showed that in low-income countries, financial barriers were the top reason cited by households for forgoing healthcare during the pandemic, while in upper-middle-income countries, COVID-19 concerns or restrictions were the top reason cited (Kakietek et al. 2022). This suggests that health system utilization rates will take longer to recover in low-income countries, as the economic fallout of the pandemic will likely linger on even after COVID-19 restrictions are lifted (Kakietek et al. 2022). Women, particularly those of lower socioeconomic status, may face greater financial barriers to accessing healthcare, as they earn less and have less control over household finances.

To accelerate recovery from the pandemic, there is a need to increase investments in essential health services and address financial barriers to healthcare. In Côte d'Ivoire, for example, the government scaled up its national health insurance program, known as the Couverture Maladie Universelle (Universal Health Coverage) (Global Financing Facility 2022). With more than 3.5 million new sign-ups between 2019 and 2021, the insurance scheme saw an 89 percent enrollment increase in three years (Global Financing Facility 2022). By the end of 2021, one-fifth of the program's enrollees were informal workers, many of whom are women, as the government began targeting the informal sector to cope with the economic fallout of the pandemic (Global Financing Facility 2022). Expanding health coverage for marginalized populations, including women in the informal sector, will reduce financial barriers to accessing care and protect them from catastrophic healthcare expenses.

Gender-Based Violence

During lockdowns, many women were confined at home with their abusers and cut off from their support systems, a situation that exposed the shocking extent of gender-based violence. According to a 2021 UN Women survey of sixteen thousand women across thirteen countries, nearly half of the women surveyed said that they or a woman they knew had experienced violence during the pandemic (UN Women 2021a). As chapters 8 and 9, from Kenya and Nigeria, demonstrate, the pandemic uncovered harmful norms around gender-based violence and reduced access to justice for survivors. Consequently, gender-based violence has been referred to as the "shadow pandemic."

Countries around the world adopted various measures to support survivors, ranging from hotlines to emergency shelters to remote social work services. In countries such as Argentina, Barbados, Côte d'Ivoire, Fiji, and South Africa, governments exempted survivors from travel restrictions and designated shelters as essential services (Staab et al. 2022). Meanwhile, in Angola, Cambodia, and Ghana, new national toll-free hotlines for gender-based violence were established (Staab et al. 2022). To meet the increased demand for shelters, Argentina, Belgium, France, and Turkey turned hotels and dormitories into temporary shelters for survivors (Staab et al. 2022). In Malaysia, service providers offered virtual social work and counseling services and used ride-hailing services to bring survivors to shelters (Joanne M. Wong, personal communication).

In addition, criminal justice systems adapted their operations to facilitate access to protection and justice during lockdowns. In Jordan, a lockdown emergency response team, spearheaded by women police officers, made home visits and safely directed victims to support services (Staab et al. 2022). To ensure that survivors could travel safely during the lockdown, police officers also accompanied survivors to the police station and court (Staab et al. 2022). In Argentina, Brazil, and the US, courts automatically renewed protection orders that had lapsed during lockdowns, while in Kenya, Mexico, and Morocco, courts permitted remote proceedings (Staab et al. 2022).

These examples are ways in which countries can ensure continuity of services for survivors during lockdowns. When declaring lockdowns, countries must act preemptively to adapt and expand services for violence survivors and not wait until reports of gender-based violence spike. Preemptive action is critical because reports of gender-based violence may not fully reflect reality due to increased barriers to reporting during lockdowns and a lag in data collection. In addition to preemptively expanding services for survivors, countries must also adopt prevention measures, such as interventions to address harmful social norms around gender-based violence.

What Enables a Gender-Responsive Pandemic Plan?

Women's participation in pandemic decision-making is vital to improving governance. Women made up just 24 percent of COVID-19 taskforce members and 18 percent of COVID-19 taskforce leaders globally, and 10 percent of taskforces had no women at all (Staab et al. 2022). As chapter 6, on China, indicates, when women and marginalized groups are not at the table, issues that affect them may be overlooked. Moreover, their exclusion raises questions about the processes by which taskforce members are selected. Women, as well as marginalized groups, have a right to participate in COVID-19 decision-making, as these decisions affect their lives and their work on the front line. The exclusion of wide swathes of the population from such decision-making not only harms democratic processes but also compromises the legitimacy of these task forces at a time when public trust is at stake. Hence, women of diverse backgrounds, as well as other marginalized groups, must be part of pandemic taskforces. In addition, these taskforces must establish channels for input and feedback so they may be more attuned to public sentiment and needs on the ground.

Political commitment is essential to enabling a gender-responsive pandemic plan and associated measures. But what political conditions enable gender-related concerns to be prioritized in pandemic responses? In their analysis of COVID-19 measures by governments around the world, the United Nations Development Programme and UN Women found three factors that were associated with increased gender-responsive pandemic measures. Countries with more women in Parliament, stronger feminist movements, and stronger democratic institutions adopted more gender-responsive policies than countries with the converse (Staab et al. 2022). Women's presence both inside and outside the government is critical, as women may face barriers to enacting change within the government (Staab et al. 2022). As such, gender equity champions from the outside can work in tandem with women's leadership from within (Staab et al. 2022). Strong democratic institutions also enable the concerns of marginalized groups, including women, to be heard and translated into policies (Staab et al. 2022).

Alongside these political conditions, gender-related data also enable a gender-responsive pandemic plan. Collecting gender-related data is not only a technical exercise necessary to develop and monitor appropriate social, economic, and health protections and responses (Rosser et al. 2021); it is also a political exercise, as decisions over what data to collect reflect the priorities of decision-makers. Moreover, data are crucial for holding decision-makers accountable. While data alone are insufficient to influence policies, without data, gender-based inequalities may be concealed, making it harder to show their magnitude and impact as well as why they warrant public attention.

Conclusion

As the chapters in this book demonstrate, the COVID-19 pandemic has disproportionately impacted women, particularly those who are poor and from marginalized groups. Many of these impacts stem from long-standing gender inequalities that the pandemic amplified. Tackling existing gender inequalities is therefore key to shielding women and other marginalized groups from the impact of future pandemics. In this chapter, we have provided examples of how some governments have taken action to address these inequities, as well as the pandemic's effects on key gendered issues. While no government response can be held up as the ideal gender-responsive pandemic plan, such examples provide a starting point to reflect on what positive developments have been seen within the COVID-19 response and what gaps remain.

Countries must act to safeguard women's livelihoods, relieve and redistribute the burden of care work, support women healthcare workers, prioritize mental health, ensure the continuity of essential health services, tackle gender-based violence, increase girls' access to education, and include women of diverse backgrounds in decision-making. Crises such as the COVID-19 pandemic provide a window of opportunity to reset priorities and adopt new approaches, an opportunity that can be seized to place gender on the policy agenda. Gender-responsive policies will not only spur recovery from the COVID-19 pandemic but will also leave us better prepared to face the next one.

References

Agency for Clinical Innovation. n.d. "Trauma-Informed Care and Practice in Mental Health Services." https://aci.health.nsw.gov.au/networks/mental-health/trauma-informed-care-and-practice-in-mental-health-services.

COVID-19 Mental Disorders Collaborators. 2021. "Global Prevalence and Burden of Depressive and Anxiety Disorders in 204 Countries and Territories in 2020 Due to the COVID-19 Pandemic." *Lancet* 398 (10312): 1700–1712. https://doi.org/10.1016/S0140-6736(21)02143-7.

David, Eden, Jonathan M. DePierro, Deborah B. Marin, Vanshdeep Sharma, Dennis S. Charney, and Craig L. Katz. 2022. "COVID-19 Pandemic Support Programs for Healthcare Workers and Implications for Occupational Mental Health: A Narrative Review." *Psychiatric Quarterly* 93 (1): 227–247. https://doi.org/10.1007/s11126-021-09952-5.

Department of Finance Canada. 2021. "A Canada-Wide Early Learning and Child Care Plan." https://www.canada.ca/en/department-finance/news/2021/12/a-canada-wide-early-learning-and-child-care-plan.html.

Flor, Luisa S., Joseph Friedman, Cory N. Spencer, John Cagney, Alejandra Arrieta, Molly E. Herbert, Caroline Stein, et al. 2022. "Quantifying the Effects of the COVID-19 Pandemic on Gender Equality on Health, Social, and Economic Indicators: A Comprehensive Review of Data from March, 2020, to September, 2021." *Lancet* 399 (10344): 2381–2397. https://doi.org/10.1016/S0140-6736(22)00008-3.

Gentilini, Ugo, Mohamed Almenfi, Hrishikesh T. M. M. Iyengar, Yuko Okamura, John Austin Downes, Pamela Dale, Michael Weber, et al. 2022. "Social Protection and Jobs Responses to COVID-19: A Real-Time Review of Country Measures." *World Bank Group*. February 16. http://documents.worldbank.org/curated/en/110221643895832724/Social-Protection-and-Jobs-Responses-to-COVID-19-A-Real-Time-Review-of-Country-Measures.

Global Financing Facility. 2022. *2020–2021 Annual Report: Putting Women, Children and Adolescents at the Center of an Inclusive, Resilient Response and Recovery*. Washington DC: World Bank. https://www.globalfinancingfacility.org/sites/gff_new/files/documents/GFF-Annual-Report-2020-2021.pdf.

Janata, Barbara, and Katherine Stewart. 2019. "Use It or Lose It: Why Taking Parental Leave Is So Important for Fathers." *Rand*. March 4. https://www.rand.org/pubs/commentary/2019/03/use-it-or-lose-it-why-taking-parental-leave-is-so-important.html.

Kakietek, Jakub Jan, Julia Dayton Eberwein, Nicholas Stacey, David Newhouse, and Nobuo Yoshida. 2022. "Foregone Healthcare during the COVID-19 Pandemic: Early Survey Estimates from 39 Low- and Middle-Income Countries." *Health Policy and Planning* 37 (6): 771–778. https://doi.org/10.1093/heapol/czac024.

The Lancet Global Health. 2020. "Mental Health Matters." *Lancet Global Health* 8 (11): E1352. https://doi.org/10.1016/S2214-109X(20)30432-0.

Morgan, Rosemary, Heang Lee Tan, Niki Oveisi, Christina Memmott, Alexander Korzuchowski, Kate Hawkins, and Julia Smith. 2022. "Women Healthcare Workers' Experiences during COVID-19 and Other Crises: A Scoping Review." *International Journal of Nursing Studies Advances* 4: 100066. https://doi.org/10.1016/j.ijnsa.2022.100066.

OECD. 2021. "Caregiving in Crisis: Gender Inequality in Paid and Unpaid Work during COVID-19—OECD." https://www.oecd.org/content/dam/oecd/en/publications

/reports/2021/12/caregiving-in-crisis-gender-inequality-in-paid-and-unpaid-work-during-covid-19_85044948/3555d164-en.pdf.

Rosser, Erica N., Rosemary Morgan, Heang-Lee Tan, Kate Hawkins, Anne Ngunjiri, Amy Oyekunle, Brunah Schall, et al. 2021. "How to Create a Gender-Responsive Pandemic Plan: Addressing the Secondary Effects of COVID-19." Gender and COVID-19 Project. https://www.genderandcovid-19.org/how-to-create-a-gender-responsive-pandemic-plan-addressing-the-secondary-effects-of-covid-19/.

Shanahan, Matthew. 2022. "The Mobile Gender Gap Report 2022." GSMA. https://www.gsma.com/r/wp-content/uploads/2022/06/The-Mobile-Gender-Gap-Report-2022.pdf.

Staab, Silke, Loui Williams, Constanza Tabbush, Camila Arza, Esuna Dugarova, Joanna Hill, and Brianna Howell. 2022. *Government Responses to COVID-19: Lessons on Gender Equality for a World in Turmoil*. New York: UN Women and UNDP. https://www.unwomen.org/en/digital-library/publications/2022/06/government-responses-to-covid-19-lessons-on-gender-equality-for-a-world-in-turmoil.

Tan, Heang-Lee, Amy Oyekunle, Uche Ralph-Opara, Erica Rosser, Rosemary Morgan, and Kate Hawkins. 2021. "How Has Nigeria Responded to the Gendered Impacts of COVID-19." Gender and COVID-19 Project. https://www.genderandcovid-19.org/wp-content/uploads/2021/09/PAC00467_Gender-and-Covid-19-Nigerias-Pandemic-Response.pdf.

UNCTAD. 2021. "How COVID-19 Triggered the Digital and E-commerce Turning Point." UNCTAD. March 15. https://unctad.org/news/how-covid-19-triggered-digital-and-e-commerce-turning-point.

UNDP (United Nations Development Programme). 2022. "COVID-19 Global Gender Response Tracker." https://data.undp.org/gendertracker/.

UN Women. 2021a. "Measuring the Shadow Pandemic: Violence against Women during COVID-19." United Nations. https://data.unwomen.org/sites/default/files/documents/Publications/Measuring-shadow-pandemic.pdf.

UN Women. 2021b. "Women and Girls Left Behind: Glaring Gaps in the Pandemic Response." United Nations. https://data.unwomen.org/sites/default/files/documents/Publications/glaring-gaps-response-RGA.pdf.

Wenham, Clare, Michelle Fernandez, Marcela G. Corrêa, Gabriela Lotta, Brunah Schall, Mariela C. Rocha, and Denise N. Pimenta. 2022. "Gender and Race on the Frontline: Experiences of Health Workers in Brazil during the COVID-19 Pandemic." *Social Politics: International Studies in Gender, State and Society* 29 (4): 1144–1167. https://doi.org/10.1093/sp/jxab031.

WHO (World Health Organization). 2018. *Mental Health Atlas 2017*. Geneva: World Health Organization. https://www.who.int/publications/i/item/9789241514019.

World Bank. 2021a. "Account Ownership at a Financial Institution or with a Mobile-Money-Service Provider, Female (% of Population Ages 15+)." https://genderdata.worldbank.org/en/indicator/fx-own-totl-zs.

World Bank. 2021b. "Account Ownership at a Financial Institution or with a Mobile-Money-Service Provider, Male (% of Population Ages 15+)." https://data.worldbank.org/indicator/FX.OWN.TOTL.MA.ZS.

12 Conclusion

Julia Smith and Clare Wenham

In this book we have brought together nine diverse case studies that narrate the experiences of diverse groups of women in the face of a global crisis. Women around the world were both central to the delivery of the COVID-19 response and disproportionately affected by its secondary effects. Lost income and opportunities, increased unpaid care work, and violence were not caused by the pathogen but occurred on account of preexisting structural inequities that pervade global political, economic, and social systems and structures. This inequality permeated global and local responses to the pandemic that, on the whole, only included gender considerations in the most superficial ways—for example, by celebrating women's work as essential (i.e., "clap for carers") but not valuing it in terms of money, protection, or resources (Harman 2021; Folbre et al. 2021). Each chapter depicts how gender roles intersected with other inequities in the home and at work to generate women's economic dependency on men, reducing their autonomy and creating opportunities for exploitation and violence during the pandemic.

This is not to say women's experiences around the world should be conflated as one and the same. Our transnational feminist perspectives speak to their heterogeneity and the importance of highlighting the localized experiences of different groups of women impacted by the same global crisis: the comparative quantitative chapter on Kenya, Nigeria, and Bangladesh demonstrates great variation of the effects of the pandemic on time use, food insecurity, and job loss across genders. Job loss, for example, has different implications in a country with strong social protection policies in places such as Canada compared to a context that does not have these, such as Nigeria. It is also important to recognize that even in a country with such protections, they are not available to all, with notable inequities related to race and citizenship, as illustrated in the chapter on Hong Kong. Social, economic, political, legal, religious, and cultural structures and institutions at the global, state, and local levels resulted in certain women having greater resources to cope with the secondary effects of the pandemic, while others face barriers accessing basic necessities and healthcare. The case studies in this book focus on how such barriers are gendered while recognizing other axes of inequality. They speak to how power relationships have been exercised, not only through coercive means such as lockdowns and police-enforced quarantine, but also through materials and ideas—for example, around neoliberal structures that determine who has priority access to vaccines and who is responsible to fill care deficits. By applying a transnational feminist analysis across a range of case studies and groups of women, the chapters in this book illustrate how dominant patriarchal, colonial, and neoliberal structures are reflected in local responses to the COVID-19 pandemic to affect a variety of women's lived experiences in ways that are both unique and share commonalities, or as we term them, "solidarities of difference."

In many countries, women are most likely to be employed precariously (Benach et al. 2016). The case studies here illustrate how such precarity, although experienced in different ways, increased women's risk of income and employment loss during crises, such as that of COVID-19. In Nigeria, informal market traders were unable to access supplies to maintain their businesses and did not have the access to credit required to weather such disruptions. In Brazil, increased precarity was associated with the loss of other forms of employment and the need for flexibility due to increased unpaid care responsibilities. In Canada, the overrepresentation of immigrant women in the food and accommodation sector—due to barriers accessing other employment opportunities as well as gender-related trends within the labor force—meant these women also faced the greatest employment losses. In Kenya, community health volunteers (CHVs) were not paid for their essential and they did not have consistent access to basic PPE or to vaccines to keep themselves safe. Such precarity is not by accident or necessity—it is created by government labor and immigration policies that perpetuate systems of colonialization and imperialism and by a global political economy of corporate privileging of profits over people.

It is this labor-related precarity that has a direct association with unpaid care. Patriarchal structures within national and global systems determined that policy levers that would facilitate women's access to paid work (such as low-cost childcare) were absent prior to COVID-19. This meant that when the pandemic hit, women, and particularly women in lower-paid jobs who work in essential services and are unable to work remotely with their children at home (who in many contexts are also most likely to be racialized), were further isolated from employment, which intersects with women's provision of unpaid care. When women living in slum communities in Brazil lost access to childcare due to school closures, they had to give up paid work. Mothers in Hong Kong struggled with prolonged school closures and their impact on professional opportunities. Case studies from China and Kenya in particular illustrated the direct relationship between disruptions in the unpaid and paid care economies. In both cases, sociocultural norms expecting women to fill unpaid care responsibilities inhibited healthcare workers from fulfilling their paid work, with implications for health system responses to crisis. A lack of accessible childcare in Canada created barriers to recent immigrant women reentering the workforce following lockdown. Neglect of maternity care in the UK meant pregnant women were forgotten in the pandemic response. Respondents in Bangladesh recognized that men's work outside the home was valued more than women's work inside the home, even though women were providing essential care. In the absence of adequate care infrastructure, women formed their own social supports. Sharing food and care responsibilities, coming together in peer support groups and advocating for their right to access basic supplies occurred in Bangladesh, Hong Kong, the UK, Kenya, and Nigeria. Chapter 11 points to how efforts to prepare for future health crises can catalyze such endeavors and buttress them with supportive policies, as opposed to exploiting and exhausting women's unpaid care labor.

Resulting income disruptions and increased care burdens negatively impacted food security for women and their families. In Bangladesh, women were more scared of starvation than of COVID-19. In Nigeria, women with disabilities had reduced mobility support and therefore reduced access to goods. Women's social positioning as being responsible for ensuring that their families were fed and cared for meant they bore the burden of trying to fill nutrition gaps, whether by going without food themselves or accessing credit informally from store holders. Interestingly, despite being disproportionately affected by income loss and food insecurity, women in Kenya and Bangladesh also took on increased income-earning responsibility. CHVs in Kenya spoke of how as the only member of their household working, they became increasingly responsible for necessities. Women in Bangladesh often became responsible for accessing credit, due to gender norms that positioned them as more reliable for repayments owing to their gendered lack of mobility. These women not only fulfilled a double shift during the crisis but also bore double the responsibility.

While states provided varying supports to mitigate financial hardship across the case studies, in all instances respondents in need faced barriers to accessing these. Women living in informal settlements in Nigeria and Bangladesh reported not receiving any support, except for sporadic aid from civil society groups. Foreign domestic workers in Hong Kong did not qualify for government financial relief because they were not citizens. Recent immigrant women in Canada could not access supports if they did not have an employment history. It is telling that, in all case studies, women with both heightened financial needs and responsibilities for others could not access pandemic response programs that were presented as assisting those in the greatest need. Chapter 11 suggests, based on evidence from other contexts, that gender-sensitive cash transfer programs might be one approach to mitigating financial insecurity during crisis.

Financial stress and uncertainty were identified as drivers of violence within households in Bangladesh, Brazil, Kenya, and Nigeria. These experiences shed light on trends from quantitative research in the same countries that indicates increased conflict within households during the pandemic (chapter 10; Wenham et al. 2022). The Nigerian and Bangladesh qualitative research in particular demonstrates how among our sampled women, pre-pandemic gender norms fostered a tolerance for gender-based violence that meant little preventative action was taken even as incidents were likely increasing. In Brazil, women spoke of how male unemployment contributed to violence, illustrating how masculine gender norms can also be harmful to women. In Kenya, CHVs discussed facing the risk of violence not only at home but also in the community, either from those they cared for or owing to perceptions that they were more likely to transmit COVID-19. There is growing literature around gender-based violence during health crises that builds on themes around financial insecurity, stress, and access to justice, as well as suggesting varying responses (John et al. 2021; Roesch et al. 2020). The case studies here indicate a need to focus on the underlying determinants that predate and then are likely exacerbated by a crisis in order to inform prevention, as well as response, strategies.

Three chapters (those on Kenya, Hong Kong, and China) describe how women staffed the front lines of the COVID-19 responses as the vast majority of healthcare workers. With the early spread of COVID-19 in China and, to a lesser degree, Hong Kong, these healthcare workers in particular risked their lives during a time when information was scarce, health outcomes were poor, personal protective equipment was scarce, and vaccines were unavailable. Evidence from healthcare workers in Wuhan, China, illustrates how the initial response was structured by gender norms in terms of who was making decisions and who was celebrated as heroes of the response (men in both cases), as well as who had to manage unpaid care responsibilities alongside increased work demands while fighting for the right to do their job safely (women). In Hong Kong, women similarly discussed having little say in decision-making around the healthcare response while providing the labor that enabled a rapid scale-up and shift in services. CHVs in Kenya were paradoxically both essential to the response, particularly in rural and informal communities, and relegated to the periphery of the health system. Despite having close contact with the illness, they struggled to access PPE and vaccines and were rarely paid even a stipend. Like the other healthcare workers, they lived with the constant fear of infecting their families and others they provided care to. These cases provide the evidence of lived experience to the calls to increase women's participation in pandemic response and health system decision-making documented in chapter 11. Women on the front lines not only deserve the right to provide input into their working conditions and be paid fairly, but often hold crucial knowledge about the effectiveness of interventions that can strengthen the pandemic response.

Healthcare workers also faced particular challenges to their mental health due to high-stress work environments and the fear of infection discussed above. Other determinants of mental health, identified across the case studies and constituent groups of women, included managing their "double shift" of paid and unpaid labor and financial insecurity, as well as loneliness and isolation when women had to stay at home while caring for dependents. In Nigeria and Bangladesh, the increase in protective measures, such as cleaning, caused anxiety around keeping families safe. In Canada, newcomer women were anxious about their ability to provide adequate home-schooling support to their children. Similarly, mothers in Hong Kong worried about their children's well-being due to prolonged isolation. Such commonalities demonstrate how women's social role within families and communities means women assume responsibility for the health and well-being of others and how, when it becomes impossible to fulfill such responsibilities during a crisis, they bear the weight of failure. Such lived experiences are further depicted in quantitative data that are particularly concerning, as they indicate that mental health continued to deteriorate two years after the start of the pandemic.

Despite the risks to mental health posed by the pandemic, most women whose experiences are recounted in these chapters did not have access to formal mental health support. CHVs in Kenya, who were not formally integrated into the health system, were not offered any wellness support. In Canada, immigrant women faced language, technical, and cultural barriers to access virtual mental healthcare. Chapter 11 indicates that such barriers are common across the globe and suggests increases in funding for mental health programs, particularly the training of mental health providers.

The chapter on the UK illustrates what happens when maternity provision is not just deprioritized but forgotten amid the pandemic response. Restrictions on partners attending births, the consequences of missed appointments, and lack of social support meant pregnant people and new parents did not get the quality of care required. In particular, the classification of pregnant people as clinically vulnerable put the onus on the individual, as opposed to the state, to ensure the health of parents and infants. Lack of clear government policies led to confusion and variation in services across the country. This lack of consideration reflects an omission of gender responsiveness within pandemic policy and planning, with the impact of this falling on the shoulders of women.

Yet we do not wish to paint women solely as victims of patriarchal structures. As transnational feminists, we are as cognizant of the variation of experience of different women as of how their gender intersects with their overlapping identities to bear inequalities, but also of the role that women play in communities and societies as advocates for change. The women we interviewed also exercised agency in trying to mitigate and overcome the gendered structural impediments that were amplified during the pandemic. The chapters demonstrate how women advocated for their rights and ensured the health and safety of their families and communities, despite the lack of policy support to do so formally. In Canada, immigrant women came together to provide mutual support during the crisis. Women healthcare workers in

China demanded equal treatment and a say in decision-making. In Brazil and Nigeria, civil society organizations, notably run by women, filled gaps in the government response. In Bangladesh, women living in slums went to great lengths to ensure their children were fed. In the UK, women shared antenatal- and postnatal-related information peer to peer through new-parent groups because of limitations of formal interaction with healthcare providers. Thus, these are case studies of resilience to the similar policies introduced in multiple governments in the face of a global crisis and struggle to change oppressive systems. Yet they demonstrate more than this—not only are women able to enact agency to improve their situations and those of their families when they are left out of the policy space by decision-makers prioritizing the "tyranny of the urgent" (Smith 2019) (in this case, controlling transmission of the pathogen), but that they assume a broader responsibility within communities. Women in each case study have shown that they will fill the gaps left by the government response, although in different ways: through mutual aid groups, community assistance, information sharing, and beyond. This speaks to broader trends across the global health space, where women provide such community functions routinely. As such, during COVID-19, the lack of government consideration of gendered effects and the needs of the most vulnerable communities may be strategic, as women are providing the solution at the community level to the gap in state provision of support (Harman 2021). The resilience, innovation and agency of women across these case studies and demographics must not only be celebrated, but supported, resourced, and centered in pandemic preparedness and response. Chapter 11 begins to sketch out how this might be achieved, including the need for political commitment to gender-responsive pandemic planning.

While we have described the common structures that disadvantage women and burden them disproportionately with the secondary effects of a public health crisis and have documented the solidarities in how women around the world in different contexts resist these, we also recognize the multiple nuanced differences among women. We have tried to emphasize and highlight these differential impacts where possible, focusing, for example, on the experiences of recent immigrant women in Canada, women living with disabilities in Nigeria, and ethnic minority women in Hong Kong. While we do not claim to be undertaking complex intersectional analyses, we do recognize the diversity of experience. We hope that by including case studies from a variety of constituent groups, identified by feminist researchers in each country as a key social community to consider, across diverse geographical locations and a myriad of states with differing governance regimes, we offer some consideration of the differing experiences around the globe. We recognize that this is an incomplete analysis and that in privileging gender as our starting point, we may have obscured other structural, racial, colonial, and neoliberal inequities that exist and are amplified during emergencies. We also recognize that this book's consideration of women exclusively also conceals the realities of those nonbinary and LGBTIQ* (Lesbian, Gay, Bisexual, Trans, Intersect, and Queer) individuals and groups living throughout a pandemic. We encourage future and further research that deepens the intersectional analysis initiated here.

Moreover, we also wish to echo our earlier consideration of our own positionality in writing this book. As researchers, regardless of the wide variety of social systems, races, geographies, communities, disciplines, and institutions, we are all privileged in many respects (although in different ways), and thus, while we all lived through the same pandemic and negotiated the realities of that within our own social and personal lives, we did not experience the pandemic in the same way as others or bear the brunt of the impacts that the women we document here experienced.

A further limitation that we wish to consider is the temporality of our analysis. The interviews that make up the data for this book took place over a two-year period, although the individual case study countries' data collection period varied (for example, Hong Kong's data collection took place within a five-month window in 2020, whereas Brazil's data collection did not start until mid-2021). Thus, the data collection periods did not necessarily overlap each other or coincide with waves of infection within communities and the associated stringency of public health measures, such as school closures and lockdowns in each location. This means two things for our analysis: first, that comparisons between case studies is imperfect, as each group of women would not have been experiencing life at the same point on an epidemic curve, not to mention the differentiation between the health and social measures brought in by governments. Second, for those interviewed in the latter stages of the research project, there would necessarily have been both more reflection back to how they experienced the initial shock of the pandemic emerging, and they also may have been managing ongoing or additional challenges that COVID-19 laid bare. For example, there would be different experiences of school closures if this was in the first wave of infection, when there remained some novelty and leeway with employers, compared to school closures that persisted into the second year (such as in Brazil) or with adjusting to the "new normal" of flexible working and finding ways of coping with the longer-term burnout that many women were experiencing, having lived through the pandemic for multiple years. We caution readers to consider this temporality when reading and reflecting on the findings.

With these limitations in mind, we believe that this book offers several novel contributions to the burgeoning landscape of research on the social effects of pandemics, and feminist global health security in particular. The first of these is simply to document the quasi-real-time effects of COVID-19 on diverse populations of women across the world, so that this can be recorded for posterity and as an evidence base to inform research and policy makers in the future about the impact of public health policy. While the ways in which women were impacted varied, depending on the context and individual attributes of the women interviewed, we highlight that the structural inequalities and drivers of oppression were globally pervasive. While previous research has identified the impacts of epidemics on women (Smith 2019; Harman 2016; Davies and Bennett 2016; Wenham 2021), these were restricted to particular national contexts. Our contribution in this way is to demonstrate that there were transnational determinants of gender inequalities whereby women suffered the disproportionate impact of the pandemic, although in different ways. Given that each country was responding to the same pathogen, and often responded with the same policy tools, this should to some extent be unsurprising.

Second, we contribute to the knowledge base that seeks to identify the cause of common, though different in type and degree, impacts of pandemic policy on women: that of global patriarchal structures (Galtung 1969; Caprioli 2005). While there are a variety of political, social, and economic structures that dominate all systems of governance and policymaking in our case studies, we argue that in each of these cases, patriarchal structures exist and influence decision-making. Accordingly, these establish traditions, institutional structures and cultural norms that, if not opposed, determine that policies implemented at a time of crisis will be gender blind, with the knock-on effect of gender-blind policymaking being that women will absorb the additional financial, social, and health costs of crisis (Wenham 2021). All public policy has unintended consequences, but as those that design policy and the crisis framing exist within a patriarchal policy environment (whether or not they are themselves men), the needs of women and other vulnerable groups are often forgotten. It is no surprise that this occurs when governance structures are themselves locations of masculinity and were constructed by men and for men over centuries and that these spaces do not facilitate more pluralistic understandings of policymaking (Tickener 1992; True 2003). While similar arguments can and have been made about the dominance of capitalist and colonial systems in policymaking, and how these in turn have shaped pandemic response, our analysis, with its focus on women's lived experiences, particularly speaks to the influence of patriarchy.

While in many locations, and during "peace-time," equality legislation and/or advisors have been brought in to try and preidentify the downstream effects of policies on particular marginalized groups, this did not appear to be the case during COVID-19 (Herten-Crabb and Wenham 2021). The age-old adage of the "tyranny of the urgent" meant that safeguarding the most marginalized fell by the wayside (Smith 2019). This has important policy-relevant ramifications and lessons for future pandemic preparedness and response efforts. Gender and intersectional responsiveness in pandemic preparedness and response cannot be an afterthought but needs to be integrated into the initial stages of preparedness and prevention, as well as design for the rapid response mechanisms, so as to ensure that women and other marginalized communities do not suffer to the extent that they have throughout this pandemic (see chapter 11). One way to achieve this is through more meaningful engagement with gender or equality advisors to mainstream policy development processes, seeking to preempt unintended consequences.

This question of unintended consequences leads to a third contribution of this work, which amplifies the recognition of the dual burden that women face in global health crises. Not only do women suffer most from the downstream effects of policies intended to stop disease, but they are the ones that in turn bear the responsibilities associated with mitigating these impacts (Wenham 2021; Harman 2021). That is, it is not by accident that gender consideration is missing from pandemic-related policy, but it may be part of the design by government decision-makers. Government policy cannot achieve everything, and administrations must decide what to prioritize. We saw this acutely during COVID-19 as governments decided on the balance between public health versus the economy. Yet it appears that few, if any, governments sought to put women and women's needs at the center of decision-making.

This may not be a surprise, in that state structures will prioritize the longevity of the state above all, but it may also reveal a broader occurrence. Were women not considered because those (mainly men) decision-makers did not consider how COVID-19-related policy might affect them? Or was it that they knew, given performative gender norms, that women would take agency to plug the gaps that the state was unable to provide (Harman 2021). In doing so, recognizing that this work and effort would be done by women, for free, governments could focus their efforts elsewhere on the response. We demonstrate in this collection of case studies that governments collectively failed to introduce meaningful policy to support women. Even when we consider the gender relations context prior to COVID-19 and analyze gender policy–progressive states, such as Canada, governments were limited in their on-the-ground implementation of support to some of the most vulnerable women (Smith et al. 2021). To that extent, a further finding is that gender relations prior to COVID-19 did not seem to affect the outcomes for women at a time of crisis.

Furthermore, we believe that this work acts as a benchmark for future research. First, we recognize that these case studies have only captured the effects of COVID-19 when it was in its acute phase of transmission and for particular communities identified as at-risk by the feminist researchers we collaborated with. The policy landscape for managing the pandemic continues to evolve in tandem with the variants that emerge. As we learn to "live with the virus," differential and new impacts will emerge that will affect women and the variety of groups of women in different locations and contexts, and these will need to be researched and analyzed over the fullness of time. Moreover, we know that many policy effects are long term, and indeed, the full extent of the impact of COVID-19 on women may not be known for many years, as the burn-out, mental health, and physical well-being may be initially masked to some extent and only become apparent at a later stage.

This research has predominantly focused on those women who have been affected by policymaking, and this has not enabled a detailed consideration of the policy process and development. Research is required on the supply side of policy and decision-making to better understand how pandemic response mechanisms were developed by governments (and nongovernmental actors) and to understand how and on what evidence decisions were made and to what extent gender played a role in this process. While we do not assume that there is one way in which each of the nine governments considered in this book developed policy, we must better understand the variety of processes, as well as a feedback loop for evidence into policy, to learn from the experience of the pandemic. We believe, however, that the case studies in this book speak to a broader phenomenon of a lack of gender considerations in public policy and particularly that of crisis management. This research would greatly benefit from collaboration and exploration beyond the landscape of pandemics and global health policy.

In closing, we note that this book is the cumulation of three years of research across multiple countries and teams. Each of the chapters is authored by women who are not only leading feminist research and advocacy in their country but who have also been living with many of the effects of the pandemic described above. We held countless meetings with children on laps (sometimes nursing), rearranged research schedules when team members had to isolate, and provided peer support when the stress of the pandemic became too much. As editors, we are immensely grateful for the perseverance and dedication of the team throughout this tumultuous time. The Gender and COVID-19 Project has provided immense opportunities for learning across contexts. We are honored to have been able to bring this learning together in this volume.

References

Benach, Joan, Alejandra Vives, Gemma Tarafa, Carlos Delclos, and Carles Muntaner. 2016. "What Should We Know about Precarious Employment and Health in 2025? Framing the Agenda for the Next Decade of Research." *International Journal of Epidemiology* 45 (1): 232–238.

Folber, Nancy, Leila Gautham, and Kristin Smith. 2021. "Essential Workers and Care Penalties in the United States." *Feminist Economics* 27 (1–2): 173–187

Harman, Sophie. 2021. "Threat Not Solution: Gender, Global Health Security and COVID-19." *International Affairs* 97 (3): 601–623.

John, Neetu, Charlotte Roy, Mary Mwangi, Neha Raval, and Terry McGovern. 2021. "COVID-19 and Gender-Based Violence (GBV): Hard-to-Reach Women and Girls, Services, and Programmes in Kenya." *Gender & Development* 29 (1): 55–71.

Roesch, Elizabeth, Avin Amin, Jhumka Gupta, and Claudia García-Moreno. 2020. "Violence against Women during Covid-19 Pandemic Restrictions." *British Medical Journal* 369: m1712.

Smith, Julia. 2019. "Overcoming the 'Tyranny of the Urgent': Integrating Gender into Disease Outbreak Preparedness and Response." *Gender & Development* 27 (2): 355–369.

Smith, Julia, Alice Mũrage, Ingrid Lui, and Rosemary Morgan. 2022. "Integrating Gender-Based Analysis Plus into Policy Responses to COVID-19: Lived Experiences of Lockdown in British Columbia." *Social Politics: International Studies in Gender, State & Society* 29 (4): 1168–1191.

Tickner, J. Ann. 1992. *Gender and International Relations: Feminist Perspectives on Achieving Global Security*. New York: Columbia University Press.

True, Jacqui. 2010. "Mainstreaming Gender in Global Public Policy. International Feminist Journal of Politics." 5 (3): 368–396.

Wenham, Clare, Michelle Fernandez, Marcela G. Corrêa, Gabriela Lotta, Brunah Schall, Mariela C. Rocha, and Denise N. Pimenta. 2022. "Gender and Race on the Frontline: Experiences of Health Workers in Brazil during the COVID-19 Pandemic." *Social Politics: International Studies in Gender, State & Society* 29 (4): 1144–1167.

Index

Page numbers followed by a *t* indicate tables; an *f* indicates a figure.

Publisher contact:
The MIT Press
Massachusetts Institute of Technology
77 Massachusetts Avenue, Cambridge, MA 02139
mitpress.mit.edu

EU Authorised Representative:
Easy Access System Europe, Mustamäe tee 50,
10621 Tallinn, Estonia
gpsr.requests@easproject.com

Printed by Integrated Books International,
United States of America